Overcoming Obesity

Overcoming Obesity

✦

Personal Insight from a Christian Physician

Jean-Ronel Corbier, MD and Michelle Corbier, MD

iUniverse, Inc.
New York Lincoln Shanghai

Overcoming Obesity
Personal Insight from a Christian Physician

Copyright © 2005 by Jean-Ronel Corbier

iUniverse books may be ordered through booksellers or by contacting:

iUniverse
2021 Pine Lake Road, Suite 100
Lincoln, NE 68512
www.iuniverse.com
1-800-Authors (1-800-288-4677)

ISBN: 0-595-34708-8

Printed in the United States of America

Contents

Preface

Having struggled with obesity for several years, before reaching my ideal body weight, I have firsthand knowledge of the challenges and difficulties confronting those that are overweight. I want to share my personal experiences in overcoming obesity. Many people who have seen the amount of weight I have lost have themselves been struggling with obesity and have tried various programs that have not been helpful. Obesity affects different parts of our body and mind. For many, overcoming obesity may seem impossible. I have decided to share my experiences and suggestions in this book so that others can gain the victory as I have.

My goal is that everyone who overcomes obesity is healed. That healing must be physical, mental, emotional, and especially spiritual. I want to educate people about what causes obesity, because many people are unaware of why they are obese. I provide simple strategies to help all persons who are obese to be free from the burden of obesity. I provide biblical principles to help others to lose weight, and introduce the reader to the RESTORATION model. This paradigm helped me, and continues to help me, overcome obesity.

Jean-Ronel Corbier, MD

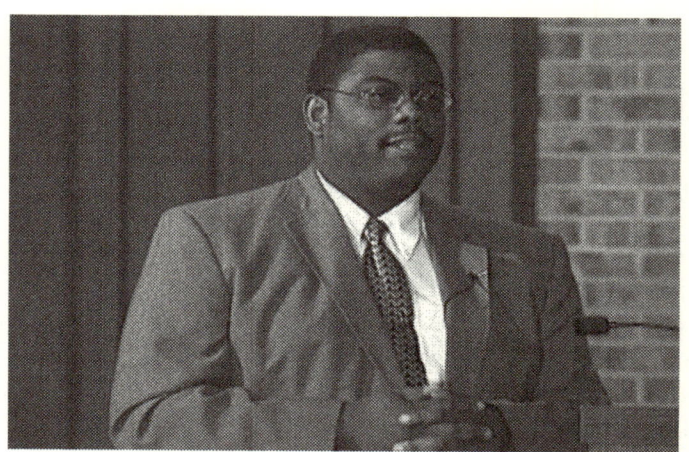

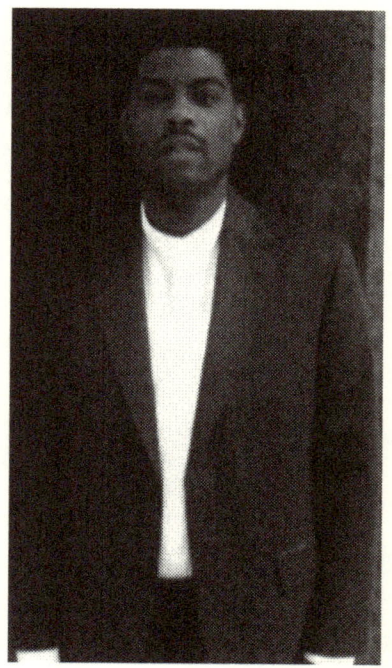

1

Introduction

I was more than 100 pounds overweight and very unhappy. As a physician I was a poor role model to my patients of good health. I would try to convince my patients and their parents of the importance of health and nutrition, but I myself was unhealthy. My body was ravaged by the co-morbid diseases of obesity: sleep apnea, insomnia, fatigue, frequent heartburn. I was often out of breath after many activities, even mild ones. The psychological ramifications of my obesity were overwhelming. My self-image was horrible. Any reference made about obesity seemed to be directed specifically to me.

I did not know what to do about my weight. How and where do I start? I was too embarrassed to ask for help. I had been obese for so long that I had little hope that I could overcome this disease. I believed that my medical practice caused my obesity, and it was just an occupational hazard. Although I knew intellectually that I was simply rationalizing, I could not help it. My thoughts were constantly about losing all my excess weight. Trying to lose weight was becoming an obsession.

Now that I have lost over 100 pounds I feel great! People who have not seen me since I lost the weight barely recognize me! I have so much energy! My heartburn, fatigue, sleep apnea, back pain and insomnia are gone. The greatest change has been to my self-esteem. I have been totally transformed into a new person, physically, mentally, and spiritually. I had to attack my problem with obesity from various dimensions. This is how I got the victory!

Obesity is a multifactorial problem. Chronic obesity is the result of many abnormal variables coming together to lead to dysfunction and disease. Genes are an important factor in the pathology that leads to obesity. But it is only *one* factor. There are people like my wife who will always be able to eat anything and never gain one single pound. Then there are those like myself, who seem to gain weight by just looking at food. Our genetic makeup determines our metabolism, which is crucial in determining whether a person is likely to become obese.

Environmental factors should not be underestimated in their contributions to obesity. Environmental stressors are perhaps more significant than the innate genetic contributions to obesity. Stress, psychology, social milieu, nutrition, personal habits, and metabolic derangements are all important aspects to obesity. But do not be thwarted, obesity can be overcome, even as I have overcome it.

2

Obesity first-hand

My slim years

In Africa I was fit, especially while I lived in Rwanda. My family moved there when I was 11 years old to do missionary work and to teach. I was not obese prior to going to Africa, but I was *heavy in build*. After a few months of arriving to Rwanda, I became thin and muscular without any effort. My lifestyle in Rwanda made it impossible for me to become overweight. Physical exercise was part of my daily routine. We walked everywhere we went since we did not own a car, including to the marketplace which was approximately five miles away. In school, we did a lot of agricultural work as part of our school curriculum. There was no television. The electricity was available only three hours daily. No one was idle or bored.

Though I had a large appetite and ate a lot, I did not gain weight. I was ridiculed because I was so thin! My diet consisted of a lot of fruits and vegetables. We grew a variety of vegetables ourselves. Everything was organic! The majority of our food was unprocessed. We drank water primarily. Occasionally we indulged in some pure fruit juices made from fruits in our garden. Sodas were simply not easily accessible where we lived. Sodas were only for special occasions.

We got plenty of rest each night as we went to bed at 9pm, when the electricity went out. We were usually tired after the day's activities and were content to go to bed. There was very little stress in my life in Rwanda. My family and I lived in a village, so we were never in a rush. It was very different from living in New York City, which is where I was born. Up until that time I lived most of my life in New York City.

Our foods were very nourishing. No pesticides were used on the fruits or vegetables. The fruits were vine-ripened. We ate a large variety of legumes, peas, beans and fruits some of which I had never heard of before. In the states, I ate all types of processed goodies like potato chips, onion rings, cookies, candy, and ice cream. Though my parents were health conscious when I was young, I was not.

In Africa, we had to eat healthy, unprocessed, raw foods. There were no other options. We had no choice but to drink water. That is what we had. Since we were very active and worked outdoors a lot, we were often thirsty, so drinking plenty of water daily was automatic. This lifestyle made it impossible to be overweight. I was the thinnest I had ever been, and would ever be, in my life. I share this part of my life because I realize that lifestyle is very important when it comes to weight management. I was fortunate back then that I was in an environment where I had no choice but to be fit. Since we did not have many options I did not get tempted to indulge in unhealthy foods or drinks. Since we did not have a car, we had to walk. Our legs were our transportation. By the end of the day we were tired from our physical labors and slept well. We expended all the calories we had consumed throughout the day.

Interestingly, when my family moved to Ivory Coast we felt like we were moving from farmland to city dwelling. The city we lived in was much more modernized than the one in Rwanda. We had electricity 24 hours a day, seven days a week. We owned a car, but not a television, though they were available. The market sold more processed foods than to which we had become accustomed. I still remained fit without trying though. We continued to eat plenty of fresh raw fruits and vegetables. We remained physically active. We chose to walk to school, even though it was several miles away. Water remained our primary beverage, although we had greater access to sodas and juices.

While living in Ivory Coast, we went on furlough (vacation) for the first time, returning to the United States. We remained in the States for 3 months. Our relatives were concerned that we appeared so thin. They wanted to know what happened to us. Immediately, they started fattening us up with food. The foods we ate were neither raw nor fresh. The foods were overly processed. We watched television and became 'couch potatoes'. We considered this as our way of having a good vacation. Our relatives felt we were 'recovering' from being too thin.

When my identical twin brother and I returned to Ivory Coast we were almost unrecognizable. Our African friends laughed at us! They could not believe what happened to us. We had gained so much weight! However, after only a few weeks of resuming our normal activities in Ivory Coast, we burned off all the excess fat. We did not make a conscious effort to do so, it just happened naturally. We simply got back to our previous routine and the weight came off quickly.

What happened to me in Africa highlights several important factors pertaining to weight balance and obesity:

1. **Metabolism is affected by lifestyle**. As an adolescent, my metabolism was probably fast anyway. But in Africa, I did things that allowed my metabolism to work optimally: eating nutritious foods such as fresh, raw fruits and vegetables and other unprocessed foods, hydration with plenty of water, daily physical activity and adequate rest. When I came to back to the States, my lifestyle changed dramatically. I put on a lot of weight *automatically*. When I went back to Africa, I again changed my metabolism, effortlessly by *automatically* returning to the lifestyle that we had previously adopted and the weight came off.

2. **Changes happen for the best or the worst.** The fact that I had a wonderful lifestyle in Africa and that I was fit, did not prevent me from gaining a lot of weight when I came back to the States. Mainly because my lifestyle changed. I was protected from obesity only as long as my lifestyle supported proper fat metabolism. Although I gained a lot of weight on my furlough, I was able to lose it again when I changed to my previous lifestyle. Although genes play a role, I believe that the majority of individuals are largely affected by their lifestyle when it comes to obesity and weight gain.

3. **Lifestyle is like a machine where all the parts are essential for proper functioning**. When one is concerned about weight loss, it is important to focus on nutrition, exercise, dietary supplements, eating habits, and stress management collectively. To only focus on one of these parts is to neglect the whole. All these factors are interrelated and directly impact each other. Remember, the whole is greater than the sum of each part.

4. **Weight management should be incorporated into your daily routine.** The goal should be to adopt a lifestyle that can be maintained permanently and one that is healthy. Do not resort to quick fixes. You may lose weight quickly, only to regain it back quickly, and usually with interest!

5. **Wellness is absolute instead of relative.** You are either well or you are not. Proper lifestyle is a *whole* package where each ingredient is important. Moreover, each element supports the other in a *synergistic* fashion.

When I lived in Africa, I had very little stress, especially compared to what I would experience in the next few years. Stress-free living is a vital part of health, wellness, and weight management. In addition to physical and mental health, my spiritual health was great. Spiritual health is important for mental health, which, in turn supports physical wellbeing.

BECOMING FAT

My journey to obesity began when I started experiencing stress, a sedentary lifestyle and consumption of processed foods. When I returned from Africa after 7 years, I eventually enrolled as a medical student at Michigan State University. Up until I started medical school, my weight was good. I did start gaining weight as soon as I returned to the States, but it was a slow, gradual process. During medical school, however, there was an exponential increase in my weight that persisted throughout medical school, residency, and worsened during my neurology specialty training. It escalated during my first few years of starting private medical practice.

In my case, everything that could go wrong went wrong. I ate the wrong foods and lots of it. I often started my day very early, sometimes at 5 am. After eating a late meal at night, I had no desire to eat breakfast. It was too early to eat anyway. I convinced myself that by skipping breakfast I could lose a few pounds. Of course, I knew that it was not healthy to skip breakfast. I knew that breakfast was the most important meal of my day. But it did not fit with my schedule. I became more sedentary. The only exercise I got was walking between the patients' rooms and along the hospital hallways. I occasionally bought exercise equipment. Unfortunately, I did not use the equipment consistently. I rationalized that I just did not have enough time for exercise. Getting started on any exercise program was hard because I was so out of shape.

My stress level was increased as only the stress level of a busy physician can be. Since I was overworked, I often chose to relax by watching television. I felt that I needed to eat something *yummy* while watching television. I could eat endlessly while I watched television. Chronic stress is an inherent part of completing medical school, residency and specialty training. Stress has many detrimental consequences, overeating is just one of them. During most of my specialty training in neurology, I worked excessively. On many occasions I would be on two phones, responding to two urgent calls simultaneously. I worked long hours. Despite the strenuous work, I enjoyed my training experience so much that I seldom minded the long hours. But there was a price to pay for working those excessive hours. Overeating became an unhealthy way to relieve my stress.

I had another problem. I did not like to waste food. Having lived in Africa, I became conscious of our tendency to waste things here in the States. When it came to food, this meant eating everything that was on my plate. There was a time that I could eat all I wanted and not gain weight. Now was *not* that time as many of the foods I found myself eating were packed with empty calories. I recall relatives that would insist that I ate all my food, sometimes against my will. I often wondered if their influence was having an adverse effect upon me. Perhaps that is why I felt I had to clean my plate completely each time I ate even if I was already full. Often there are psychological influences that affect our eating habits.

Everything in my life had begun to conspire to transform me from being healthy and fit to being corpulent and out of shape. I might have escaped the problem of obesity if I ate the right foods, or perhaps if I remained physically active. I might even have been protected against obesity if I did not have to deal with chronic stress. With *all* of the above problems mounting each year, however, I had no chance. I was doomed. My fate was sealed. I also did not have 'slim genes' to depend upon.

I NEED TO LOSE WEIGHT ASAP

I cannot think of one advantage to being fat. I can think of countless reasons why being obese is problematic. In my case, I appeared healthy superficially. I had many health problems though. I did not sleep well because I snored, had reflux and insomnia. This also affected my wife's quality of sleep. I ate late at night and had to take antacids nightly to get me through to the next morning. My poor sleep caused excessive daytime sleepiness (hypersomnolence). Driving long distances was hazardous. I was often out of breath, even for non-strenuous activities.

My wife, who is a physician, kept giving me advice regarding what I should do to lose weight. I knew everything that she said was true, but felt powerless to comply. My twin brother, who is also a physician, reminded me that I could become a diabetic if I did not lose weight. I had significant truncal obesity, which put me at serious risk for diabetes. Thinking about the health ramifications of my obesity brought me great trepidation. In addition to diabetes, I thought of cardiac problems, endocrine abnormalities, impaired immune function and other health problems that could only lead to one eventuality, a premature death.

As an obese person the psychological ramifications were the most difficult for me to confront. My self-esteem suffered immensely. Not only was I a physician, but I always spoke to my patients about wellness and proper lifestyle. What type of example was I for my patients? I had a hard time counseling my obese patients to lose weight, when I needed to do the same thing. Being obese gave me a feeling of inadequacy that was almost unbearable.

I was also vexed spiritually. Being overweight meant that I was intemperate and lacked self-control, a glutton and on the wrong path. How could I serve God effectively when I, His temple, my body, was overweight? Was I violating the commandment that says: "though shalt have no other gods before me"? Perhaps food had become an edible god for me. Although I knew that God still loved me, I felt that I was not presenting myself to God in an acceptable way. I was not a good representative of God to others. I knew that I could not serve Him as well as I could if I were fit in body, mind and spirit. I felt it was time to ask God for help.

3

How I lost 100 lbs and Kept it off

PREPARATION PHASE

Preparation is very important in any weight loss program. One has to really want to lose weight and be prepared to do whatever it takes to do so. In addition, one has to be mentally prepared. It is important not to set yourself up for failure. One has to set goals, plan well and engage in a routine that is practical long-term. In my case, I wanted to choose a program that I knew would work for me. I did not want to do something that would be too difficult, expensive or time-consuming. The first thing I did was to imagine what life would be like if I were thin and at my ideal body weight. For a few seconds I experienced immense joy at the thought of what my life would be like if I were very fit. The joy was so intense that it was almost tangible. The goal seemed a bit unrealistic though.

I decided to fast. For four days I ate nothing. I only drank water. The main purpose of the fast was to ask God for strength. I needed to make a commitment and obtain stamina. I needed to persevere. I absolutely did not want to fail in this endeavor, and did not trust my own strength to become successful. During my fast, I prayed frequently, asking God for help. If God would hear my cry, the battle would be won. Interestingly, after a few days of fasting, I was so hungry that I longed for the time when I would be able to eat anything I desired. This allowed me to get a fresh start to eating properly. It was as if my taste buds had a chance to reset themselves.

INDUCTION PHASE

After my fast, prayer, and meditation, I was finally ready to start. My plan was to eat the right types of foods, in the right amount, and at the right time. I decided to drink plenty of water. I designed an exercise program that was fun and that I could do long-term. Initially, I tried the treadmill. I was faithful with using the treadmill for several weeks, but decided that I would be more comfortable walking each morning instead. The problem was that I felt that I needed to walk for at least one hour to get the right amount of exercise needed. This was based on the fact that I did not want to walk very fast and I wanted to also use the time I was walking as my time of daily prayer and meditation. At first, it seemed that walking for an hour was not a practical goal since I wanted to do it very early every morning. My work day usually starts very early. I did start walking, 15 minutes at first, then 20 minutes, then 30 minutes. Eventually I ended up walking 2 hours each morning. I awakened at 3 o'clock in the morning to reach my goal. Walking 2 hours in the morning and starting my day at 3am fueled my desire to reach new spiritual heights during my morning devotion, prayer and meditation.

Walking very early in the morning has allowed me to have a spiritual experience that has been nothing less then transformative. I have been able to appreciate the beauty of the starry sky. I began to study nature. This helped me mentally. Walking was a good way to relieve stress, ponder on the previous day's experiences and plan ahead for the next day. Walking forced me to drink more water and helped my bowels to function better. I slept better. In short, walking became an indispensable part of my day. By walking I got my exercise, prayer, meditation, relaxation, and many other benefits. I found that I was able to work more efficiently. I was able to come home earlier. I also went for late afternoon walks and walks on the weekend with my family. That improved our family time. Weekend and afternoon walks allowed me to receive sunlight. Sunlight is important for mood, boosting the immune system, and vitamin D formation.

I had to make some important changes when it came to my eating. I decided to never skip breakfast since breakfast is the **most** important meal of the day. To accomplish this, I had to eat lightly at night, and as *early* as possible. This meant that since I spend a good portion of the night with a relatively empty stomach, I would be hungry by morning during which time I would be able to *break the fast* or eat breakfast. I decided to drink plenty of water, at least 80 ounces of water daily. I drank water constantly between patients.

I started taking dietary supplements using a system called *Glycolean*. This provided me with glyconutrients, minerals, vitamins, antioxidants and various other nutrients that support fat burning and are natural. This system also allowed me to find out about low glycemic foods. Low glycemic foods do not elicit a large insulin release when consumed. When you consume high glycemic foods a large amount of insulin is released which leads to fat storage. I viewed the supplements as an adjunct of an overall wellness and weight loss program.

After doing the above for several days, I had mixed emotions. It seemed like I still had a very long road ahead. A few weeks after starting my regimen, I was beginning to loose weight when a patient said I appeared to be gaining weight. These types of comments at the early phase of my weight loss journey were distracting, but I knew I had to move forward toward my goal. While it felt like I had a marathon ahead of me, I believed that the victory was already won. I was pursuing a routine that I could follow with little stress and that would lead to a radical transformation in me. I was thrilled!

MAINTENANCE PHASE

Losing weight is one thing. Keeping it off is another. A few years ago, when I was in my pediatric residency training, I had decided to go on a raw diet for one month. I only ate raw fruits and vegetables and drank water. I exercised daily. At the end of the month, I lost 40 pounds, only to gain it back *with interest* shortly thereafter. I did not want the same thing to occur again. I wanted to lose weight and keep it off! What I found is that by persisting with my program, my metabolism has increased, and become more efficient. I still face temptations, but the battle is won! The greatest challenge comes when my daily routine is broken, like when I travel. Since I do not want to regress and gain the weight back, I always ask God for strength during my daily walks. Fortunately, my metabolism has improved and several things are built into my daily routine to help me maintain my weight loss. I take the stairs instead of the elevator, drink plenty of water, and eat nutritiously. These things have allowed me to maintain my ideal body weight.

4

Significance of obesity

According to the CDC (Center for Disease Control), the definition of obesity in adults is a body mass index (BMI) of greater than 30. The BMI also called the Quetelet Index, is calculated based on your height and weight, and is highly correlated with direct measures of body fat in most populations. Being overweight is defined as having a BMI of 25-29.9. The rates of obesity are increasing worldwide. The World Health Organization (WHO) stated in its report <u>Obesity: Preventing and Managing the Global Epidemic</u> that "without societal changes, a substantial and steadily rising proportion of adults will succumb to the medical complications of obesity…the spectrum of problems seen in both developing and developed countries is having so negative an impact that obesity should be regarded as today's principal neglected public health concern". Tobacco is currently the number one cause of premature death in the United States, but obesity is quickly catching up to it. "Being overweight or obese may soon cause as much preventable disease and death as cigarette smoking", said Surgeon General David Satcher. Some estimates state that obesity accounts for 7% of total health care costs in the United States. A goal has been established by health authorities to decrease the incidence of obesity to less than 15% prevalence by the year 2010. The incidence of obesity has increased in the United States from 22% to 30% between the years 1988 to 2002. The incidence of obesity in diabetics has increased to 54% in the same amount of time. Even as little as a 10% weight loss can lead to an improvement in health, and a reversal of many of the adverse effects associated with obesity. In the United States the economic impact of obesity has been estimated to have been more than $110 billion in 2000. Obesity is more common in people of lower socioeconomic status worldwide. The tendencies of obesity are greater in African-American women than Anglo-American women regardless of the economic class. However, obesity is more common in Anglo-American men compared to African-American men, with socioeconomic class not being a significant factor.

The first step in treating obesity is in finding a definition. In order to determine if someone meets the qualification for obesity, you must calculate his or her BMI. The BMI is determined by dividing an individual's mass in kilograms by their height in meters squared. A person's BMI is not affected by their age or gender. Obesity is related to genetics, metabolism, society, behavior and culture. Stated simply, obesity is the result of a greater intake of calories than those expended. To affect weight loss one must *expend* more calories than they have consumed. There are also some theories that obesity may even be related to viruses. People often state that their obesity is due to a 'glandular problem', or hypothalamic disorder. Hypothalamic obesity is generally rare. It may be caused by trauma, tumor, inflammatory processes, surgery on the posterior fossa, or increased intracranial pressure. Medications can also cause weight gain, but not usually to the point of obesity. Occasionally obesity *can* result from chronic high dose corticosteroids though.

Over 15 million people in the United States suffer with type II diabetes mellitus. There is a 40% increased incidence of diabetes for those who are over weight. In both adult men and women there is a correlation between obesity and major depression. Many diseases have been shown to be related to obesity and the lack of exercise: hypertension, stroke, thromboembolic disease, cancer, sleep apnea, gallbladder disease, kidney stones, osteoarthritis, dyslipidemias, musculoskeletal disorders, gout, and type II diabetes mellitus. The hyperinsulinemia seen in patients with obesity is thought to lead to the formation of calcium stones through the increased excretion of calcium in the urine. Also, it has been found that having a large body mass can increase the excretion of uric acid and oxalate. This thereby will increase the risk of oxalate kidney stones forming. Obesity also negatively affects pregnancy, labor and delivery. Excess abdominal girth is an independent risk factor for increased morbidity apart from obesity.

Types of cancer related to obesity:

Breast

Ovarian

Prostrate

Colon

In obesity there is also an entity called the **metabolic syndrome**. The hallmark of this condition is insulin resistance. The National Cholesterol Education Program

Adult Treatment Panel III has defined criteria for this condition. People with this condition have increased visceral fat. Obesity causes an increase in the size and number of fat cells (adipocytes). There is hypertrophic and hypercellular obesity. In hypertrophic obesity the fat cells are enlarged. Hypercellular obesity means a greater number of fat cells. Hypercellular obesity is usually present when obesity begins during childhood, which is the time of cellular differentiation and development. Hypercellular obesity also tends to be more severe, with a BMI usually greater that 40. The different types of obesity are important in showing how complex obesity is, and how it affects all persons differently.

Metabolic syndrome is defined as 2 or more of the following:

Central adiposity

Hypertension

Fasting hyperglycemia

Diabetes mellitus

Hypertriglyceridemia

Low high-density lipoprotein (HDL) cholesterol

5

Childhood obesity

"A special characteristic of obesity development in childhood is its dependence on the actions of *others* to create the circumstances that cause it or cure it" (italics added) Editors' Overview of the Conference on Preventing Childhood Obesity, Pediatrics 2004. The WHO (World Health Organization) estimates that about 17.5 million children are overweight worldwide. Childhood obesity is defined as a BMI greater than the 95th percentile, while being overweight is defined as a BMI over the 85th percentile. There are some concerns that the BMI may not be an accurate measure to determine obesity for children and adolescents across different ethnic groups. The BMI is more sensitive than specific, which may lead to some children who are obese not being included in the general definition.

One might assume that children born large for gestational age (LGA) would be more likely to become obese later in their lives. However, studies suggest that LGA infants have greater proportional lean muscle relative to their body fat. SGA (small for gestational age) infants have a larger proportion of fat. The studies therefore suggest that an adult who was SGA may be more likely to have an increased health risk of certain conditions such as obesity, hypertension, and type II diabetes. If there is a rapid increase in weight gain in the first year of life, the likelihood of later development of obesity is increased, especially for SGA infants.

Although the studies are not definite, there is evidence that breastfeeding may protect against the development of obesity in later life. It is not certain if breastfeeding is protective because it may affect later food preferences or if the relationship is due to maternal feeding practices. But it is worthy for practitioners to continue to emphasize the need to breastfeed, especially up until the first year of life. Of course it is important to emphasize to breastfeeding mothers that the quality of their milk will affect the infant's growth and development.

Most causes of childhood obesity are *not* genetic, but are due to a sedentary lifestyle and poor diet. The diet of obese children generally will consist of high fat, high calorie, and low fiber foods. One factor for practitioners to consider is that obesity due to excessive caloric intake tends to encourage an increase in stature, whereas those children who are obese from endocrine diseases usually do not have a concomitant increase in height. A study presented in Pediatrics 2001 suggested that the earlier onset of puberty in children might be related to the increase of obesity.

If we hope to decrease the incidence of adult obesity, we need to address the expanding problem of childhood obesity. Approximately 25% of children are obese. Because obese children become obese adults, it is very important to try and target obese children as early as possible. Studies are showing that infants born to mothers who were obese at the time they became pregnant are at an increased risk for also becoming obese later in their lives. This is an important reason why our goal should be to change lifestyle habits in children in the formative years of their lives. While only about 15% of adults report being obese when they were children, almost 50% of children who are obese will become obese adults.

For children, the goal is often not to cause weight loss, but to slow down the acquisition of further weight. Therefore, allowing the child to 'grow' into their weight. As the child's linear growth increases their weight should ideally be maintained and not increased. A child will need approximately 1 ½ years of linear growth to compensate for every 20% excess amount of weight above their ideal body weight. Children tend to have a steady decrease in their BMI until approximately 5-7 years of age. At that time they begin to experience an increase in their BMI. Some researchers postulate that the earlier a child experiences an increase in their BMI, or rebound in adipose tissue deposition, the higher the likelihood that the child will develop obesity later in life. What we do know is that the influences upon a child between the ages of birth and 7 years have long-term consequences for the impact of obesity upon their future life. These influences may be environmental, psychological, or medical.

It is important that children not form an abnormal ideal of their body image. This could lead to even more profound problems with eating, and ultimately affect their self-esteem. A child's self-esteem determines the relationship between obesity and the possible manifestation of depression. Obese girls are more likely to be depressed and anxious opposed to boys. Obese girls are also reported to have a higher incidence of suicide attempts. Both Anglo-American and African-American girls from lower socioeconomic status homes reported more suicide attempts because of weight problems, and admitted to having symptoms suggestive of an eating disorder.

When managing a child who is obese it is necessary to make changes that impact the entire family opposed to singling out the affected child. Parental obesity is a strong determinant of childhood obesity. Maternal obesity is more influential upon the child than paternal obesity, meaning a child is more likely to become obese if the mother is also obese opposed to the father. Obese mothers have a 4x risk of having obese children compared to non-obese mothers. Studies also show that maternal food preferences during pregnancy will affect the food preferences they make for the infant postnatally. We need to continually emphasize that improving the diet of the entire family is what is needed. What children eat is determined by what the parents purchase. So again, the parent's level of commitment is paramount.

It is helpful for the family to eat meals together at the dinner table, and not in front of the television. Watching television is a strong predictor for the onset of obesity. Many researchers recommend decreasing television viewing to less than 30 minutes daily. Not only should television use be decreased, but the amount of time on computers or with computerized games should be decreased also. Limiting the amount of time spent watching television, videos and playing video games has been shown to decrease the BMI in children. Once an infant is weaned from the breast or bottle, milk should be *completely* removed from the diet. The amount of fruit juice and sodas should be decreased also, or even completely eliminated. Fast food should be consumed no more frequently than once a month, if not less often. Highly restricted diets are not recommended for children, except in rare circumstances where the child's health may be jeopardized and even then it should only be done under the supervision of a qualified medical professional. Infants should be encouraged to walk more, instead of being pushed in strollers by their parents. Even worse are parents who carry children that are able to walk on their own. Less than 50% of all children receive daily physical education classes through the school system. So it is important that parents incorporate some form of physical exercise into the routine of children in the home and not rely on the school system to provide this needed component to the child's health.

The emphasis must be placed on parental education. The parents need to encourage a healthy food environment in the home. Parents need to model these good eating behaviors in front of their children. They also need to teach their children how to make good food choices when the children are away from home and not under the parents' supervision. One way this could be done is by having the child buy groceries and plan a meal for the family. It would also be helpful to allow the child to prepare the meal. The preparation of healthy, inexpensive, simple meals is an invaluable skill which will greatly help the child throughout their life.

Parents should be cautioned to not use food as a reward or a form of comfort. A child should not be forced to consume food when they are not hungry. Many of us remember being forced to 'clean our plates' when we were young. It is important to teach children not to waste food. But a more effective way of demonstrating this principle would be to not prepare so much food, and only place a small amount of food on the child's plate. You can always add more if the child is still hungry. More nutritious desserts should be consumed. Fresh fruits make a delicious and nutritious dessert. If parents are not knowledgeable about these things they should consider participating in a cooking class, perhaps the entire family could attend.

Parents need to be role models for physical exercise also. This may prevent the need for more parental control over eating habits which could be detrimental psychologically. Medication is currently not recommended for the treatment of children with obesity. Currently, gastric bypass is usually reserved for medical emergencies in children with life-threatening complications from their obesity. Some believe that gastric bypass surgery may be a safe weight loss alternative for teens who have been unsuccessful in losing weight by other means. It is recommended that the procedure be reserved for adolescents with a BMI greater than 40, however. A psychological assessment is also recommended to be obtained in surgical candidates for gastric bypass. The long-term requirements of dietary restrictions and vitamin/mineral supplementation must also be explained to the adolescent and the parent. A study reported in Pediatrics, July 2004, looked at laparoscopic gastric bypass surgery for severely obese teens. The criteria was the presence of a BMI of 40 or greater, skeletal maturation (13 years of age or older for females and 15 or older for males) and having obesity-related conditions "that might be remedied with durable weight loss". Several patients have done well with gastric bypass, but the risks of serious complications including death must be highlighted. Both parents and patients must be informed of the need to adhere to strict nutritional guidelines and physical activity following the surgery lifelong.

Many children, if supported by their parents, can have a change in lifestyle that can avoid the need for surgery. As mentioned previously, after surgery the patient must adhere very strictly to nutritional guidelines. Nutritional and lifestyle changes then are important whether a person decides to have a surgical operation or not. So families need to be reminded that there are no 'quick fixes', and that nutritional interventions are required regardless of the decisions made for other treatment options. Many teens that are obese are consuming foods that may also adversely affect their behavior, mood and cognition. The changes that are beneficial for weight loss may also be beneficial for improving their psychological and mental health as well. Obesity in teens as in other age groups may in some cases be related to psychosocial factors. These should always be identified and treated appropriately. Examples would include depression, anxiety disorders such as obsessive compulsive disorder (some have a compulsive need to eat), and related disturbances.

All children and adolescents who are obese need to have a complete and thorough physical examination at least annually.

Children Learn What They Live

If a child lives with criticism, he learns to condemn.
If he lives with hostility, he learns to fight
If he lives with fear, he learns to be anxious and insecure.
If he lives with pity, he learns to feel sorry for himself.
If he lives with ridicule, he learns to be shy.
If he lives with shame, he learns to feel guilty.
If he lives with encouragement, he learns to be confident in himself and his abilities.
If he lives with tolerance, he learns to be tolerant of others.
If he lives with praise, he learns to be appreciative.
If he lives with acceptance, he learns to love.
If he lives with approval, he learns to like himself.
If he lives with recognition, he learns that it is good to set goals for himself.
If he lives with security, he learns to have faith in himself and in other people.

Author unknown

6

Genetic and hormonal aspects of obesity

Scientists have identified single gene mutations that can cause severe obesity, although these cases are rare. Genes that code for leptin, leptin receptor, POMC (pro-opiomelanocortin), PC1, and MC4R can sustain mutations that can lead to obesity. Leptin is secreted by adipocytes. It binds to receptors on the hypothalamus. This leads to the stimulation of POMC production, which produces PC1 and alpha-MSH. Alpha-MSH binds to MC4R receptors in the hypothalamus, which in turn can curb food intake. The most common form of monogenic obesity is mutations of the MC4R gene. The frequency of this genetic defect is about 5% in the population. Genetic causes of obesity can be from a deficiency of leptin. Supplementation with leptin in these situations causes weight loss. A defect in the leptin receptor can cause severe obesity. People with this condition do not respond to leptin of course because the disorder is with the *receptor* for leptin. Then there is a defect in the melanocortin receptor and POMC a defective formation of that can also cause obesity. Finally, there can be a disruption in the control of the differentiation of fat cells by the peroxisome proliferators-activated receptor (PPAR) or the prohormone convertase-1 (PC-1) gene. PC-1 defects must be combined with a defect of another gene, though, for obesity to occur. Congenital forms of obesity associated with a genetic syndrome are more common than single gene defects.

Medical syndromes associated with obesity:

Prader-Willi

Bardet-Biedl

Alstrom

Angelman

Borjeson-Forssman-Lehman

Wilson-Turner syndromes

Obese individuals, interestingly, do not have a lower amount of leptin, but may have too much leptin. This in turn can result in a condition of leptin resistance. The receptors 'turn off' because of the over abundance of leptin to which they are exposed. The genetic component of obesity is yet to be clearly elucidated. Once we understand more about the role genes play in obesity the more able we will be to affect appropriate therapies to eradicate this condition. Meanwhile, it is important to re-emphasize that the majority of the afflicted individuals with obesity have no genetic component. Obesity is still primarily a condition of too many calories consumed and too little expended. Lifestyle and dietary changes are still the most important component to treatment.

7

Psychosocial and behavioral aspects of obesity

It is unfortunate but true that people are more understanding of a person who is obese because of a medical condition than from just having a problem with controlling appetite. The public disapproval of obese people leads them to be stigmatized. This public apathy can affect the psychological health of those that struggle with obesity, and only compound their level of stress. Obese persons are at a higher risk for body image distortions and binge eating. Because obese individuals are more likely to diet, they are more likely to suffer adverse psychological distress from their dieting. Studies may not show a relationship between obesity and psychological health, but we do know that depression is associated with dissatisfaction with body appearance. And if a person regains weight quickly following recent weight loss (weight cycling) they are more likely to experience psychological distress from this recurrent cycle of weight gain and loss.

Behavioral modification is the application of techniques to overcome habits that inhibit changes in lifestyle. Behavioral modification involves various techniques. It rests on the principle that changing behavior can affect weight, that behaviors are learned, and that long-term behavior changes involve changing one's environment. Despite the varied factors which affect obesity, behavioral modification focuses on current behaviors.

Behavioral Modification techniques:

1. Self monitoring

2. Stimulus control

3. Behavioral contracting

4.   Cognitive restructuring

5.   Stress management

6.   Relapse prevention

7.   Social support

Any behavioral modification program should involve: emphasis on eating break-fast, eating small frequent meals, eating slowly, not purchasing high caloric foods and keeping a food diary. Many believe that behavioral modification in combination with dietary intervention is the preferred method of treatment for obesity. One of the most effective behavioral approaches to weight loss management is a food diary. This allows a person to directly see the behaviors and activities that affect their eating patterns. This tool can also help to establish goals regarding needed dietary interventions. This tool can also provide an individual with some immediate feedback as to their progress, which can be encouraging. This provides the individual with insight into their eating behaviors. A person's ability to maintain a food diary is a strong predictor of long-term weight loss. By teaching children and adolescents to take responsibility for their own eating habits by keeping a food diary they are encouraged and strengthened psychologically. And, ultimately, those youth who do accept this responsibility will be more successful in maintaining a balanced weight.

Children and adolescents seem to be more successful with behavioral management for long-term successful weight loss compared to adults.

Individuals should be encouraged to identify environmental triggers to their eating habits. Those patterns can be changed only once they are identified. So, if a person realizes that they eat whenever they watch television, then television viewing time should be decreased. This person should also consider not having easily available snacks in the home so that the tendency to snack is curbed. A person may not be as likely to snack if it involves a longer preparation time. The goal is to positively change behaviors to a new, more desirable environment.

A behavioral contract is another effective behavioral modification tool. It involves two people, a practitioner and the individual wanting to change a behavior. The behavioral contract should be *specific* about the behavior that needs to be changed and the *consequences* of success or failure. The rewards and penalties need to be agreed upon by both parties. The contract is a form of commitment that the person struggling with obesity makes to themselves and their caregiver. This makes the obese person responsible to himself and his practitioner for adhering to the rules that have been established. It can be a way to get support in contractual form to assist a person in their goal to lose weight.

In cognitive restructuring an individual is encouraged to examine how they think about things, most importantly their obesity and future weight loss plans. A person's perception of himself will affect his ability to lose weight and how he perceives his weight loss attempts. A pessimistic attitude can interfere with any efforts at weight loss. A person needs to understand his thinking patterns to obtain better insight over how he views himself, and ultimately control himself so he can better understand his illness. Only by having good self-awareness will a person be able to improve their health.

It goes without saying that stress contributes to illness, and obesity is no different. When a person who is struggling with obesity learns how to deal with the stressors in his life his endeavors to lose weight are more likely to succeed. Stress leads to relapses in weight loss, and results in weight gain. Most people know the types of situations which are most likely to lead them to relapse in their weight loss efforts. We need to, therefore, prepare ourselves for these relapses to prevent them from leading us on a long downward spiral toward weight gain. Instead, we want to find supportive people to help us in being proactive in *preparing* for the expected stressors which can cause us to relapse. The more social support a person has in their efforts to lose weight the more successful their weight loss will be, and the longer they will be able to keep the weight off. The support should come from inside and outside the home. The family can be supportive by including themselves in the lifestyle changes that are required, to support the person trying to lose the weight. Peer support can help people realize that they are not alone in their struggle with good weight management. It is often more helpful to speak with a non-family member about the stress we experience daily, and discuss those things which cause us to fail in our efforts towards weight loss. Speaking with someone who has actually experienced the feeling of being obese can be enormously validating and successful.

Stress is a part of life that we need to prepare for because it is not a question of <u>will</u> stress come but <u>when</u>.

8

Nutrition and weight control

The word diet comes from the Latin word "diaita" which means "manner of living". One needs to change their *style of living* in order to effect and maintain weight loss. Some people even advocate avoiding the word diet all together because of the negative connotations associated with the word. A change in diet and exercise is necessary to maintain a person's ideal body weight and should therefore be in a form that is tolerable to the person.

People afflicted with obesity need to *expend* more calories than they *consume*. The majority of obese persons will need to decrease the amount of calories they consume in their diet to effect a change in their weight. The National Heart, Lung and Blood Institute (NHLBI) recommends a low-calorie diet (LCD) to include 1000-1200 kcal for women and 1200-1500 kcal for men. This dietary recommendation proposes that with these adjustments a person can achieve a loss of weight of approximately 8% in a year. This weight loss should also be accompanied by a decrease in abdominal circumference. This is significant because abdominal girth can increase a person's risk of cardiovascular disease. Very low calorie diets (VLCDs) are not recommended. They include a daily amount of 800 kcals, and are usually given in a liquid-diet formulation. VLCDs require supplementation with vitamins and minerals to satisfy the nutritional inadequacies inherent to these diets. People on VLCD are, unfortunately, at an increased risk of gallstone formation. Low fat diets are not proven to decrease weight loss anymore effectively than simply reducing the overall caloric intake. Low carbohydrate diets initially cause weight loss through the loss of water. This weight unfortunately returns when the diet returns to its previous state of carbohydrate consumption. Low carbohydrate diets may also limit fiber intake, which can lead to constipation, not to mention the deficiency of other vitamins, minerals and electrolytes. A vegetarian diet has been shown to have the lowest caloric intake. The NHLBI recommends an LCD and increased physical exercise to produce and sustain weight loss. This should also lead to a decrease in abdominal girth and subsequent improvement in cardiorespiratory status.

Binge eating is a condition where a person eats a large amount of food in a short period of time. BED, binge-eating disorder, is a condition where a person experiences recurrent episodes of binge eating with associated feelings of distress. By definition BED occurs at least twice a week for at least 6 months and the eating usually occurs in a period of less than 2 hours. Affected persons tend to have a poor self image. These individuals do not meet the criteria for anorexia nervosa or bulimia. They are often overweight or obese, but some may be normal weight also. They generally do not engage in purging or fasting and do not have the abnormal perceptions of their body image as seen in other eating disorders. Up to 25% of persons who are obese engage in binge eating. Individuals affected by BED are more likely to report a history of childhood abuse. Individuals who engage in unhealthy forms of dieting such as fasting, vomiting, purging, or diuretic/laxative use have higher levels of depression and anxiety. Healthy weight loss behaviors, such as exercise, are more likely to improve the psychological well-being of obese individuals. Another eating disorder common with obese people is called night-eating syndrome. This is a situation where about 25% of a person's daily calories are consumed in the evening. Individuals with this condition experience sleep disturbances, and occasionally sleep apnea.

A change in diet can help prevent heart disease, cancers, stroke, hypertension, and type II diabetes mellitus. A person's fat intake should not constitute more than 30% of total caloric intake, with 55% complex carbohydrates, and 15% from protein. Researchers at the Mayo Clinic have found that excessive amounts of fatty acids are toxic to the liver. A condition called NAFLD (non-alcoholic fatty liver disease) is surpassing other liver diseases in occurrence. NAFLD is related to a diet high in fats. Almost 2/3 of obese persons have NAFLD. The adolescent diet constitutes mainly refined carbohydrates (simple sugars and sweeteners). Their intake of complex carbohydrates, fiber and good fats is limited. People who are overweight eat less fiber than lean people. Because of the safety of dietary fiber and its ability to help with weight loss, it should be part of any weight reduction diet.

Calories from foods:	Calories for diet:
Fats=9kcal/g	Fats= 30%
Carbohydrates=4kcal/g	Carbohydrates= 55%
Proteins=4kcal/g	Proteins= 15%

A moderate caloric-deficit diet involves just reducing the amount of calories a person takes without making a significant change in the type of foods that are eaten. Enough food is eaten to maintain the person's present weight. This is determined by calculating the amount of energy a person expends each day. The level of physical activity that a person engages in each day is also determined. If a person eats enough to maintain their present weight and then if they increase the level of their physical activity, they can lose weight. Remember, in order to lose weight you must use more energy (calories) than you consume (eat). This is of course easier said than done though.

Glycemic indexing is a process where a determination is made as to how quickly a certain food elevates the release of insulin after it is consumed. Glycemic indexing can be a useful tool for dietary management. High glycemic foods (potatoes, white rice and white bread) are easily digested and cause a rapid increase in plasma glucose. Low glycemic foods (fruits and vegetables) are digested slowly and have a slower rise in blood glucose. High glycemic foods elevate fasting triglycerides more than lower glycemic foods. High glycemic diets can lead to a lower HDL (high density lipoproteins) level. HDL is the protective lipoprotein. It is good to have a high HDL and low LDL. Incidentally, fish oils lower triglyceride levels also.

Alcohol provides unnecessary calories while consuming needed nutrients, and should therefore be avoided.

During weight loss, people need to make sure they are taking a vitamin and mineral supplement. The National Center for Health Statistics collected data which purports to show that there may be a relationship between low calcium intake and obesity. It is, therefore, prudent to recommend that calcium supplementation be provided, up to 2000gm/day if possible. All persons desiring to lose weight should consume 8-10, 8 ounce glasses of water daily. The amount of water consumed should be increased according to the level of physical activity one engages in.

Daily intake of fiber should be increased. Total dietary fiber intake should be upto 25gm/day. Fiber can alter bile acid metabolism and decrease cholesterol synthesis. The fiber curbs appetite and decreases food intake in overweight persons. Cereal grains, fruits, vegetables, dried beans, peas, legumes, guar gum and mucilages are examples of viscous fibers. Guar gum, psyllium, and pectin can lower LDL. Cereal fiber is best at decreasing the risk of myocardial infarction, while fruits and vegetables are best at decreasing stroke risk.

Take home messages:

1. Consider the caloric value of food choices.

2. Observe food composition.

3. Read labels carefully.

4. Purchase food cautiously.

5. Avoid high caloric foods.

6. Increase water intake.

7. Decrease portion sizes.

8. Avoid drinking alcohol.

It is disturbing that reports often state that a toddler's most commonly reported vegetable consumed is French fries or fried potatoes. The Feeding Infants and Toddlers Study (FITS) found that about 10% of toddlers were consuming candy daily, almost a fourth drinking sweetened beverages, and over a fourth eating some form of junk food. Children who participate in the WIC (Women Infants and Children) program are more likely to consume fruit juices, desserts, sweets, and less likely to eat natural fruits. No difference in vegetable consumption was appreciated though between children who participated in the WIC program and those who did not. Obviously there is a problem with what parents are feeding their children. Parents are not being provided with the information needed to make the best nutritional choices for their children. Given the impact of obesity upon our society it seems that the government needs to make a greater effort to dispense useful correct information regarding nutrition.

"Most people do not consume an optimal amount of all vitamins by diet alone...it appears prudent for all adults to take vitamin supplements." JAMA, June 2002.

VITAMINS

Vitamins are substances necessary for humans to carry out normal metabolic functions. They are generally only required in small amounts. Vitamins usually have to come from sources outside of our bodies as our bodies usually cannot make these substances. Vitamins work by different mechanisms. Some vitamins act as cofactors in chemical reactions, while others may work on specific receptor sites.

Vitamin A helps to maintain the function of bones, skin, reproduction, embryonic development, the immune system and vision. Vitamin A is a fat-soluble vitamin. Retinol esters and carotenoids are major dietary sources for vitamin A. A good source of vitamin A is egg yolks, organ meats, and *fortified* milk.

Thiamine is vitamin B1, a water-soluble vitamin. It acts as a cofactor and assists in the action of decarboxylation and transketolation reactions. It should be noted that people with a high metabolic rate from physical exercise or people who mainly consume carbohydrates have higher thiamine requirements. Good sources of thiamine are yeast, nuts, rice, wheat, cereal grains and legumes. Thiamine is destroyed by heat. Excess amounts of thiamine are excreted through the urine.

Flavin mononucleotide and flavin adenine dinucleotide are the physiologically active forms of riboflavin. Riboflavin is vitamin B2. These substances are nucleotides involved in mitochondrial oxidation-reduction reactions. In the intestines riboflavin is phosphorylated to flavin. Only small amounts of riboflavin are stored. Riboflavin can be provided in eggs, enriched cereals and grains, green vegetables, and meats. The excess amounts are excreted in the stool and urine.

Nicotinamide adenine dinucleotide (NAD) and nicotinamide adenine dinucleotide phosphate (NADP) are the physiologically active forms of niacin, or nicotinic acid. Niacin is vitamin B3. The dietary source for niacin is actually the dinucleotides. The nucleotides are hydrolyzed in the small intestines. Tryptophan is another dietary source of nicotinic acid. Many types of bread are enriched with niacin. Animal protein, fish, eggs, cereals, and green vegetables, and legumes are sources of vitamin B3 also.

Vitamin B6 is a term used to describe three substances: pyridoxine, pyridoxal, and pyridoxamine. Pyridoxal phosphate is the physiologically active form of the vitamin, and functions as a cofactor. Pyridoxine is available is cereals, legumes, vegetables, eggs, fish, and meats. It is degraded by heat. Its absorption occurs in the gut.

Vitamin B12 is also called cobalamin. The cobalamins contained in meat, fish and dairy is the main dietary source for people. However, there are sufficient amounts of vitamin B12 in legumes also.

Vitamin C refers to compounds with the activities of ascorbic acid. The human body does not produce Vitamin C, it must be supplied. Vitamin C strengthens the immune system, helps with the absorption of iron, maintains skin tissue, and destroys free radicals. Vitamin C regenerates vitamin E more effectively than lipoic acid, helps in the production of collagen, prevents the oxidation of lipoproteins, and protects against cataract formation. Vitamin C also helps to preserve the energy producing capacity of the mitochondria. Vitamin C is in many fruits and vegetables. Good sources of vitamin C are oranges, citrus fruits, potatoes, strawberries, tomatoes and broccoli. It is destroyed by heat and alkalis. It is absorbed in the intestines. Excess ascorbic acid is excreted in the urine. Studies have shown that those who supplement their diet with vitamin C live healthier and longer lives.

Vitamin D refers to steroid compounds involved in the regulation of calcium and phosphate in the body. The active form of vitamin D is calcitriol. Vitamin D acts as an antioxidant. Vitamin D decreases the activity of free radicals, effects immunoregulation, and helps to prevent osteoporosis. Cold water fish, *fortified* milk, cod liver oil, and liver are good sources of vitamin D. If a person is able to receive optimal exposure and amounts of sunlight, then dietary supplementation of vitamin D is unnecessary.

Vitamin E is a group of fat-soluble substances that act as scavengers for free radicals. Alpha-tocopherols are the most important of these substances. Vitamin E can destroy free radicals, supports the immune system, and helps to prevent arterial clots. Vitamin E can help protect people from diseases like Alzheimer's disease, heart disease, and several types of cancer. Exercise depletes the body of its antioxidants. Vitamin E can destroy free radicals, but then becomes a free radical itself that can be recycled. It is recycled into an antioxidant by vitamin C and CoQ10. Vitamin E travels in the body via lipoproteins. Lipoproteins are produced in the liver. It also protects the lipoproteins from oxidation, which is believed to be the first step towards atherosclerosis formation in the arteries. Caution should be exercised with using vitamin E in people taking antithrombotic and antiplatelet agents. Vitamin E may also decrease the efficacy of statins. Vitamin E is found in eggs, vegetable oils, nuts, nut butters, barley and green leafy vegetables. Alpha-tocopherols are especially prevalent in vegetable oils.

Biotin is a cofactor of four carboxylases. Bacteria in the human intestines synthesize biotin. Biotin is present in several types of food products. The amount of biotin which comes from gut flora opposed to that from the diet is unknown. But biotin is found in barley, egg yolks, avocado, bread, broccoli, chicken and fish.

Vitamin K is fat-soluble. Vitamin K assists with the synthesis of blood clotting factors in the body, and may also help to support bone integrity. Gut bacteria also synthesis vitamin K in the intestines of humans. A good source of vitamin K is cabbage, cauliflower, leafy greens, cereal, soy beans, and vegetables.

The folates are pterydine compounds. They assist in cell growth and division. Dietary sources of folate are cereals, leafy vegetables, legumes, organ meats, and orange juice.

ANTIOXIDANTS

Vitamins C and E, glutathione, lipoic acid and Coenzyme Q10 (CoQ10) are antioxidants. Vitamin C and E are obtained through the diet, but not produced in the body. The other three antioxidants are produced in the body. The levels of these antioxidants decline as we age, that is why supplementation is needed. The antioxidants work synergistically. The antioxidants work at preventing the loss of other antioxidants through oxidation. The antioxidants work by strengthening the immune system. Antioxidants govern cell growth, and can prevent cell mutations.

Lipoic acid is the most versatile and powerful of the antioxidants. It potentiates the action of the other antioxidants. It may protect against strokes and heart disease. Lipoic acid can increase the levels of glutathione in the body. It also removes toxins from the body. It can recycle antioxidants such as vitamins E and C, CoQ10 and glutathione. Alpha-lipoic acid can be effective in preventing early diabetic glomerular injury.

CoQ10 is a fat-soluble molecule. It is actually a co-enzyme, which means that it works in conjunction with an enzyme to produce cellular reactions. CoQ10 works in the Krebs cycle to produce ATP. It therefore, is necessary for the production of energy in the body. CoQ10 is present in all cell membranes. The largest amounts of CoQ10 are found in the mitochondria of the cell. That is where energy production occurs. It works in conjunction with vitamin E to protect the cell membrane from attack from free radicals. CoQ10 is converted to ubiquinol, which prolongs the action of vitamin E. CoQ10 has been documented to be an effective treatment for heart failure, angina and high blood pressure. In Japan, CoQ10 has been used to treat and prevent heart disease. It can revitalize neuronal cells, regenerate vitamin E and treat Alzheimer's, Parkinson's disease, gum disease and possibly breast cancer. It offers protection from UV radiation also. The level of CoQ10 decreases with age. CoQ10 may decrease the efficacy of chemotherapeutic drugs and radiation therapy. It can also lower the INR in patients taking coumadin. It is made in the body, but can be obtained from seafood and organ meats.

Glutathione is the most abundant antioxidant in the body. It is water-soluble and is actually produced in the body. The three amino acids that form the structure of glutathione are: glutamic acid, cysteine and glycine. Glutathione helps store and transport amino acids. Glutathione is not very effective in oral supplementation. N-acetyl-cysteine (NAC) enhances brain glutathione production. It acts as an antioxidant, and decreases the formation of the free radical nitric oxide. After the age of forty the production of glutathione in the body declines. Certain substances can deplete the levels of glutathione in our bodies. These substances include: cigarette smoke, nitrate in luncheon meats and alcohol.

Minerals

Chromium— lowers blood glucose

Lowers HbA1c

Improves insulin sensitivity

Magnesium—increases the release of insulin

Its deficiency is associated with increased insulin resistance.

Selenium—   supports the antioxidants.

Carotenoids—an antioxidant.

Daily recommendations:

CoQ10 30mg

Lipoic acid 1200mg (will help boost glutathione levels)

Calcium 2000gm

Chromium 200mcg

Iron 10-20mg

Magnesium 40-400mg

Selenium 45-200 micrograms

Vitamin A (retinol) 900-2300mg

Vitamin B1 (thiamine) 1.5mg

Vitamin B2 (riboflavin) 1-1.8mg

Vitamin B3 (niacin) 15-35mg

Vitamin B6 (pyridoxine) 1.5-2mg

Vitamin B12 (cobalamin) 2.5-3mg

Vitamin C (ascorbic acid) 75-100mg (1-2gm in diabetics)

Vitamin D (calcitriol) 5-10 micrograms *or 10 minutes of sunlight*

Vitamin E (tocopherols and tocotrienols) 25-500IU

Vitamin H (biotin) 25-100 micrograms

Vitamin K (phylloquinone) 10-30 micrograms

Vitamin M (folic acid) 500mg/day

Zinc 5-15mg

ESSENTIAL FATTY ACIDS

Linolenic and linoleic acid are important EFAs in prostaglandin formation. Linoleic acid is a precursor for PG1 (prostaglandin 1). Diets rich in vegetables, nuts, seeds, and fish are good sources of linolenic and linoleic acids. They lead to the formation of PG1 and PG3. Animal fats, dairy products and animal protein are sources for PG2 (prostaglandin 2). Primrose oil, borage oil and black currant seed oil are rich sources of linoleic acid. Flaxseed oil contains linolenic acid. Linoleic acid may decrease fat deposition, increased lipolysis and increased fat oxidation. It should be refrigerated, as should all the liquid oil supplements. Dietary fats and essential fatty acids from the omega-3 and omega-6 groups decrease the inflammatory process in the body.

GLYCOPROTEINS

Mannose, galactose, xylose, fucose, N-acetylglucosamine, N-acetylgalactosamine, and sialic acid (N-acetylneuraminic acid) are monosaccharides primarily used in the body for cellular function. Glycoproteins are a combination of sugars and proteins. Glycoproteins on the surface of the cells help with cell-to-cell communication. Glycoproteins are also on the surfaces of other molecules, which circulate in the blood stream. The body preferentially absorbs these molecules from the diet, instead of the laborious process of manufacturing them through enzymatic processing. However, if your diet is deficient in these substances your body has no choice but to manufacture them.

9

Exercise and weight control

The CDC (Center of Disease Control) and the American College of Sports Medicine (ACSM) recommends that all adults receive >30 minutes of exercise daily. Almost 30% of adults are not involved in any form of physical activity. Those who are most likely to be inactive are women, minorities, and the less educated from lower income homes, obese persons, and older persons. Half of the individuals who begin an exercise program will stop in 6-12 months. Exercise should be considered a **planned, structured repetitive activity** in order for it to improve a person's fitness. Less than a quarter of the people over 65 years in age are involved in any physical activity. It has been shown that **just walking** can decrease mortality.

People have three primary ways in which they burn energy: food utilization, resting energy expenditure (REE) and physical activity. REE account for 60% of our daily energy consumption, but is relatively similar between obese and non-obese persons. Only by increasing one's physical activity level will energy expenditures (calories burned) outpace energy consumption (calories eaten). The lack of exercise will increase a person's risk of cardiovascular disease three-fold. The combination of the lack of physical activity and obesity together will lead to a decrease in the *quality* of life.

EXERCISE:

Increases HDL level in men

Benefits women when their weight becomes constant, not during active weight loss

Helps to lower triglycerides

When comparing people who use diets to lose weight and those who use exercise, the amount of weight loss is comparable. The difference, however, is that those who exercise also benefit from greater total fat reduction and increased cardiovascular fitness. This would support a combination program of both diet and exercise. Especially as we age, exercise is important to maintain our weight. Adolescents and children may benefit from suggestions to *decrease* sedentary activities instead of encouraging *intense* physical activities. By giving them the choice to choose their preferred activities, they are more likely to choose those pursuits that hold more interest for them. Therefore, giving more chance for long-term pursuit of those activities opposed to the more sedentary activities they were engaged in previously.

When beginning any exercise program consider the intensity and the amount of activity the program involves. The intensity of physical activity is expressed as a metabolic equivalent (MET). A MET is measured as the ratio of the metabolic rate for an activity divided by the resting metabolic rate. 1 MET is equivalent to 1kcal/kg body weight per hour. There are graphs to tell you how many METs are involved in a given activity. Pedometers can be used to measure the amount of walking a person does daily. This is another way to record how many calories are being expended, or the amount of energy that is burned during your activities.

Either resistance or strength training can help a person to lose weight while also improving the cardiovascular system and endurance. Strength training also helps to increase lean body mass. The ACSM recommends that diabetics participate in 30-60 minutes of low to moderate intensity physical activity at least twice weekly. Any physical exercise program should involve 5-10 minutes of warm-up and cool-down activity.

Another form of exercise is called lifestyle activity. This involves changing the way you do things in your everyday life. An example is taking the stairs at work instead of the elevator. Parking farther away in the parking lot to get to the grocery store can increase your physical activity. Lifestyle activity has proven to be an effective form of weight loss. It may be more practical for those people less inclined to participate in a more structured physical activity program. The important thing to remember is that there are several options for exercise. It is imperative that you choose the program which is most practical for you and your lifestyle. An excellent program is no good if you will not be able to adhere to the program. If you do not know what will work for you, consider asking a medical practitioner, a physical trainer, or a gym/fitness club.

10

Alternative therapies and weight loss

Almost half of all adults have tried some form of alternative therapy in trying to achieve health and wellness. More and more parents are trying herbal medications for themselves and their children. Managed care is even making alternatives therapies more available to patients. Physicians need to be aware of the varied treatments available to patients, and try to recommend those most appropriate to their patients. The use of herbal medicines and alternatives therapies has greatly increased in the last decade. Herbal medicines alone are a billion dollar industry which is only growing in the United States.

The Dietary Supplements Health Education Act of 1994 (DSHEA) allows consumers to purchase herbal products without a prescription. It also provided for the formation of the Centers for Dietary Supplement Research in Botanicals supported by the National Institutes of Health (NIH) through the Office of Dietary Supplements and the National Center for Complementary and Alternative Medicine. This allows for clinical and basic research investigations on dietary supplements for the prevention of various diseases. The goal is to provide the public with useful information on the potential benefits of botanical products. The Food and Drug Administration (FDA) has not released any regulations regarding product labeling, manufacturing processes and quality control measures for herbal preparations, however. The European market more closely regulates the sale of herbal products overseas. They are regulated similar to pharmaceuticals in Europe. The amount of substance in some herbal preparations is also questionable. Samples from the same company may often vary in their concentrations even between different bottles. It should be remembered that herbal supplement manufacturers are not allowed to claim to "treat, prevent, cure, mitigate, or diagnose a specific disease". The DSHEA does not require testing for safety or efficacy of herbal products. There is no product purity standards established for herbal products either. The other complication is that manufacturers of herbal products are not required to report incidents of adverse outcomes to the FDA. Anyone who wishes to report an adverse event associated with an herbal product can contact **MedWatch at 800-FDA-1088** or the national **Poison Control Center at 800-222-1222**.

It is important to remember that herbs are drugs, and must be used with caution. Often when people are using herbs they are doing so without the assistance of a physician or medical practitioner. They are in fact *self-medicating*. With this in mind it is important that the consumer educate themselves as much as possible about herbs, and their potential side effects. Herbs work because of their inherent chemical strengths. These strengths can also be harmful if used improperly or in the wrong situations. It is noteworthy that children metabolize medications, even herbal ones, differently than do adults. Because they have proportionally larger livers for their bodies, they detoxify substances differently than adults. They also have a growing developing neurological system which is more sensitive to toxins and chemicals.

Ephedra alkaloids and herbal forms of caffeine (guarana, ma huang or gotu kola) are popular supplements for weight control and energy boosters. There is a synergistic relationship between ephedrine and caffeine. Herbal products use ephedra, which is a combination of related compounds, with ephedrine being the most biologically active of the substances. In common pharmaceutical products ephedrine is used in a more purified, potent form, along with caffeine. It is believed that caffeine helps in weight loss by increasing oxygen consumption and fat oxidation. Ephedrine elevates oxygen consumption but does not increase food intake, thereby leading to weight loss. Ephedrine works by activating the beta-3 adrenergic receptors. The activation of these receptors leads to tissue thermogenesis, which causes the rise in oxygen consumption. Ephedra has been reported to cause high blood pressure, heart palpitations, liver disease, and strokes. Ephedra and caffeine can cause euphoria and a 'natural high' which can make them popular with adolescents and adults. They are touted as being 'safe' weight loss products.

Green tea is commonly used in Asia. Green tea contains caffeine. Black tea is more commonly used throughout the world. Black tea is formed by allowing green tea to oxidize. The catechins in the green tea convert to theaflavins. The catechins are a family of compounds that are flavonoids, which include the strong antioxidant epigallocatechin gallate. Green tea extract is better than caffeine at stimulation of thermogenesis in adipose tissue.

Herbal products for weight loss:

Ephedra

Caffeine

Green tea

Citrus aurantium

Capsaicin

Garcinia cambogia

Guar gum

Glucomannan

Garlic is one of the most commonly used herbal preparations in the US. Garlic has been shown to decrease the level of cholesterol. Garlic can interact with certain drugs, however, like warfarin and chlorpropamide. Garlic is often used to treat diabetes and obesity. Soybeans contain a large amount of isoflavones. They are also high in soluble fiber and decrease the elevation of blood sugar by delaying the absorption of glucose. Plant sterols have been shown to decrease LDL levels. So it is obvious that herbal or nutritional therapies can be of assistance in helping with a weight loss regimen. But the contribution of these products should not be overestimated. It is still recommended that they be used with a program of exercise and dietary intervention.

CAM stands for complementary and alternative medicine. Because almost half of all Americans have used some form of alternative therapy at some time, it is imperative that medical practitioners ask patients about possible CAM therapies they may currently be using. Often, though, patients are hesitant to reveal the CAM therapies they are using, fearing reproach and chastisement by their medical caregivers.

CAM therapies:

Acupuncture

Ayurveda

Biofeedback

Chiropractic

Homeopathy

Hypnotherapy

Light therapy

Magnetic therapy

Music therapy

Naturopathy

Osteopathy

Sound therapy

Things to remember about natural therapies:

1. 'Natural' does not mean *safe*.

2. Do your research and get all the information you can.

3. Obtain expert guidance if possible.

4. Herbs may have side effects, just like medications.

5. The quality of herbal preparations can vary.

6. **All** your medical care givers (including medical doctors) need to know which herbs you or your child is receiving.

7. **All** your medical care givers need to know about any 'alternative therapies' which you or your child is receiving.

8. Many alternative therapies have licensing organizations, so you may and should verify the credentials of your practitioner.

It should be remembered that many of our most common medications were originally derived from plants (i.e. salicylate, cocaine, and digitalis).

11

Drugs, surgery and weight loss programs

WEIGHT LOSS PROGRAMS

Americans spend more than $30 billion annually on weight loss treatments. Before beginning a weight loss program any obese individual should have a full physical examination by a medical professional, especially if they have a significant medical illness, i.e. diabetes mellitus. Experts do not recommend losing more that 2lbs/week. The initial goal of a weight loss program should be to decrease one's weight by 10% in the first 6 months of the program. Frequently meeting with others for encouragement in your efforts to lose weight is especially important in the first 6 months of a new program. During active weight loss a person may need to see their physician as often as monthly, especially if they have concomitant health problems. Remember that there are no 'quick fixes'. Weight loss must involve lifestyle changes to be effective and long lasting.

Any weight loss program to be successful will require the participant to be fully motivated. Any weight reduction program should involve behavior modification, diet/nutrition education, and information about exercise programs. Many different forms of weight loss can be employed. It has been proven though that by incorporating several different types of programs at the same time you can greatly improve your initial weight loss chances and increase the length of time the weight stays off. Studies show that we need to **emphasize fitness**, not simply weight loss. Diabetes Care, in their 2004 article, showed that men who are obese but moderately fit had a lower death rate than normal weight unfit men. Studies also show that people over 80 years old who are fit, can be in better shape than their unfit counterparts who are 20 years younger. These studies tell us that we should encourage fitness over weight loss.

Before beginning a weight reduction program consider:

1.   Raising the issue of healthful eating.

2.   Determine your readiness.

3.   Assess your current eating habits.

4.   Determine areas that need help.

5.   Set realistic goals, long-term and short-term.

6.   Obtain counseling, if needed.

Before a child is involved in any weight management program, one must assess the state of readiness or cooperation from the family. Ask the family how concerned they are with the child's current weight, what they believe needs to be done, and what can be done, and what changes *they* can make to affect those changes. Children and adolescents may do better in a treatment program in which a parent is also involved. Please note that older people do not lose weight as readily as younger person's involved in comparable programs.

PHARMACOLOGICAL TREATMENTS

There is currently a lot of research investigating medications to treat obesity. Pharmacological agents should still be used in conjunction with diet and exercise regimens though. The long-term safety of weight loss medications has not been proven, and these drugs must be continuously scrutinized. Most persons regain their weight after discontinuing their weight loss medications, however. Obesity requires a **lifestyle change** that must be continued to maintain weight loss. Along with anti-obesity drugs there are now fat substitutes that are being used in food substances. One example of these food additives is Olestra. One must be aware that these food additives may affect the absorption of vitamins and minerals in the body.

There are also studies being done to investigate the possibilities of using gene therapy to fight the battle against obesity. Researchers at the University of Florida are looking at gene therapy targeted at the POMC (pro-opiomelanocortin) gene. The researchers have discovered that the POMC gene has helped obese rats to lose weight compared to those rats not injected with the POMC gene. This could be significant in helping obese persons who may be genetically conditioned towards obesity. Other genetic research is targeted toward discovering what signals may be present in our bodies to commit some cells to become fat cells. At Johns Hopkins University researchers have found a protein called BMP4 which can induce stem cells in mice to become adipocytes.

SURGICAL OPTIONS

There are various surgical options that have been used including liposuction and gastric bypass surgeries to cause weight loss. Who are candidates and what are the pros and cons? There has been some discussion about whether liposuction helps correct the metabolic derangements associated with obesity. Although a significant amount of fat may be removed during the process, it is not generally believed that liposuction leads to an improvement in the metabolic abnormalities such as insulin resistance and elevated cholesterol associated with obesity. There are several different forms of gastric bypass surgery. They differ in how much bowel may be removed and where the actual anastomosis is placed in the bypass surgery. The significance can determine not only the side effects or complications of the surgery, but also the need for dietary supplementation. Presently, all persons undergoing gastric bypass surgery will require dietary restrictions and vitamin supplementation for life. The outcomes in regards to weight loss are good, but the complications are real and serious.

12

Reversing obesity with the RESTORATION model

Are you having problems losing weight? Does it seem like you are fighting a hopeless cause? Let me share with you a model that will help with more than weight loss. It will show you how you can be transformed and totally restored. We have developed a RESTORATION model of health and healing that is dynamic, comprehensive, and integrative. The model as it pertains to obesity, which I consider an illness, and various other health challenges, is explained as follows:

- The RESTORATION model is based on a deep understanding of biopsycho-sociospiritual factors.

  - Instead of focusing on just biological causes of illness and dysfunction, it also looks at psychological, social and spiritual causes. Biological distur-bances can affect our mental well-being and disrupt our social milieu. This can adversely affect our spirituality. The reverse is also true.

  - A primarily spiritual problem can affect every aspect of our existence including ones that are biologically-based. A person who is failing to lose weight by focusing primarily on biomedical factors may be more successful if pychosociospiritual factors are considered. Although a greater acceptance and appreciation of psychosocial factors has occurred in the past few years, spiritual concerns are poorly understood and often ignored.

  - Spirituality is crucial when it comes to health problems, a perfect example being that of obesity. Spiritual virtues such as faith, humility, love, peace and joy can be thought of as **spiritual vitamins** that may be deficient and cause problems.

- Negative attitudes and emotions such as chronic fear, guilt, resentment, revenge, and pessimism are examples of **spiritual toxins** that provide the need for spiritual detoxification and cleansing.

- Negative emotions may do any or all of the following:

  - Interfere with sleep
  - Cause gastrointestinal symptoms
  - Cause hypertension (high blood pressure)
  - Cause headaches
  - Cause anxiety symptoms
  - Cause mood disorder
  - Cause chronic syndromes
  - Cause fatigue
  - Impair memory and concentration

Negative emotions can also lead to such devastating illnesses like strokes and heart attacks, if there are additional risk factors. Apart from the physical effects of obesity, there are emotional factors as well that can have serious consequences. Secondary emotional factors also develop that only complicate the situation further.

If instead of chronic fear, guilt, or other negative feelings someone decides to place their faith in God with the belief that He is all powerful, you can see how that person's blood pressure could decrease. He may gain peace, happiness, joy, and become empowered to reach his objective of losing weight.

Faith is vital. It is interesting to note that Christ, when He was on earth, accomplished numerous miracles. He often said "your faith has made you whole". Faith must be important if Christ repeatedly made this statement. Faith is more than belief. It is an active, dynamic process that allows an individual to have access to healing that would otherwise not be possible. My belief is that through prayer, fasting and faith, Christ was able to make me whole. He did so by renewing my mind, granting me the will and time to exercise daily, and consistently supplying the special insight and strength needed to totally alter my lifestyle gave me what I needed to succeed. During this process, He gave me peace, trust, and the realization that my weight loss was inevitable and just a matter of time.

- The RESTORATION model is holistic.

  - Full restoration is only possible when all the components that may be contributing to illness are taken into consideration. This includes biological, psychological, social and spiritual factors. In addition, total RESTORATION as far as biology is concerned, requires an approach that works with, instead of against, the body. Suppressing a symptom with drugs is not the same as correcting a nutritional deficiency or avoiding food toxins that may be causing the problem in the first place.

  - Imagine a person with chronic hypertension, lupus, diabetes or migraine headaches being told: 'Your condition is chronic, and life-long. We do not know why you have this problem. You will need to take pills for the rest of your life. You must be compliant with this medication', as opposed to a person who is told 'There are various problems that may be contributing to your condition including diet, lifestyle, stress and genetic predisposition. While we may not be able to alter your genes, there are many ways that we can help to encourage your body's natural healing mechanisms or *the doctor within* by the grace of God. God is able to help you, and I will do what I can to support you'. Everything the body needs for proper functioning such as proper nutrition, proper hydration with water, exercise, good social and spiritual support, adequate rest, and temperance is vital not only for maintenance of optimal wellness but also for the re-establishment of total health.

- The RESTORATION model is etiologic-based.

  - Complete return to health cannot occur unless the underlying problem is addressed. The body has an innate healing mechanism that usually allows it to carry out its own curative action, independent of medical intervention. A good example is a viral upper respiratory or ear infection for which an antibiotic (useless against viral infections) is prescribed for two weeks. After two weeks the person gets better because the viral infection is terminated and overcome by the immune system. It so happens that the antibiotic was prescribed for the same length of time. A misinformed person might sing the praises of a drug that did nothing towards healing them. People must realize that illness is not a medication deficiency problem. A headache is not caused by ibuprofen deficiency any more than heartburn is caused by a ranitidine deficiency. Headaches can be caused by numerous factors, often nutrition and lifestyle related, that could be easily corrected without medication. This is the same with obesity, there are a variety of factors that are involved and must be addressed in order for complete healing to occur permanently.

- What about genes? Genetics are important in the manifestation of most illnesses, obesity included. But genetics is simply one contributing factor. At most, genes may cause vulnerability in an individual, but with proper lifestyle, attitude, nutrition and spiritual strength, the genetic vulnerability will remain simply a genetic vulnerability. Some people have to struggle more than others when it comes to weight issues. Unlike my wife who can eat whatever she wants, whenever she wants and remain thin, it would seem that just looking at food makes me gain weight. Despite the fact that there are obese individuals on both sides of my family, I was able, by using the principles of the RESTORATION model, to lose 100 lbs!

- There is no sickness gene. There are no genes that exist to cause disease. Instead, when genes are abnormally expressed or mutated they can code for proteins that can lead to metabolic derangements resulting in illness. We should be careful not to judge people because we do not know what genetic susceptibilities may be affecting a person's ability to lose weight or to become healthy. If you consider the illnesses that bring people to the doctor's office or hospital, the actual cause of these diseases is often nutrition, lifestyle or stress related. Statistically then, addressing these issues thoroughly should result in restoration of health for many.

- The RESTORATION model is curative.

  - Instead of palliative, our model is restorative. It is based on the understanding that total healing is possible, even if it requires a miracle. Divine intervention may be the only way to be healed in certain cases. This model places no limitations on the possibility of healing, even for refractory cases. Healing is not predicated on diagnosis, chronicity, cause, genetic vulnerability, or virulence of the infection. Instead, the level of faith, prayer, and God's willingness to intervene are the most important factors. This model is one that brings hope and comfort.

  - Although a cure is never impossible, a cure may not always be God's will. In a broad spiritual context, sometimes good may come from a person's afflictions. It may provide good for the person or others around them. The illness may only be temporary. If someone who is going through a chronic illness understands the RESTORATION model they would be equipped to face the illness with a positive attitude and hope. Hope, by itself, may help them become healed.

- You must take responsibility for your actions always. Remember that the consequences for your choices may last a lifetime. Violating simple health principles may lead to an illness, with secondary, tertiary and quaternary problems that can further compromise your health. Divine intervention should never be expected, if there is willful and persistent violation of health laws.

The RESTORATION model is complete. In order for its application to have positive effects, it must be completely understood. All of the principles in the model are important. The model cannot be effective if only a few principles are applied and others are ignored. These principles work together. They are all interrelated. Applying all of the principles will cause synergistic results.

You are not _saved_ by your diet, but you are _healed_ by it! Practical application of the RESTORATION model: Prescription for health and healing

RESTORATION can be used as an acronym that describes specifically the steps needed to obtain a full return to health:

R—RENEWAL

"Create in me a pure heart, O God, and renew a steadfast spirit within me."
Ps 51:10

When it comes to chronic obesity, no real improvement can occur without the renewal of mind. This is where everything begins. There needs to be a renewal of attitude and approach toward wellness. Understanding that obesity is a conquerable problem will _already_ initiate some very positive changes toward weight loss.

A renewal entails a complete makeover, a total alteration. This is a type of change that can only come from God. Even with individuals who possess an inner strength to change, that willpower and inner strength are a gift from God. Unfortunately, many individuals with chronic obesity feel, helpless and hopeless. Such individuals are in desperate need of total renewal of mind and body. If you have a problem with obesity, start with the recognition that there is a problem, which must be corrected. No matter how severe your weight problem, the following applies:

- Ask God to bring a total renewal of your mind and body. God is the author of all good things and is willing to help you.

- You must surrender to God entirely. Follow God's laws, religious and health laws.

- Start exercising faith.

- A renewal requires being humble. Your pride may interfere with many things, including divine intervention.

- Total renewal requires having a forgiving heart. The inability to forgive yourself and others can affect your mental health. Good mental health is a requirement for successful weight loss.

- Become committed to a full lifestyle change.

- Avoid procrastination. Don't start tomorrow. Get started today!

- It is important to remain focused, and not become distracted by negative thoughts. Instead of focusing on your present shortcomings, contemplate you future success.

E—EXERCISE

"Six days you shall labor and do all your work"
Exodus 20: 9

Exercise is vital. You must take time to exercise. There should be absolutely no excuse when it comes to exercise. Whether you have a very hectic schedule or are bed-ridden, you should still exercise. You may need to start slowly and discuss an exercise program with your physician if you are unfit or have heart disease, but you must exercise. By exercising, you turn on a powerful system that does the following:

- Burn fat calories.

- Speed your metabolism.

- Restore your energy.

- Improve your quality of sleep.

- Help your bowels to work better.

- Detoxify your body by eliminating harmful toxins.

- Enhance your immune and endocrine (hormone) systems.

Exercise is a good way to fight stress and improve mood. Because consistency is essential, I recommend a very simple exercise that can be continued throughout life with multiple benefits that has worked for me:

- **Walk** for 1 hour, early, every morning at approximately the same time each day.

- Walk at a pace that is convenient and comfortable.

- If possible, choose a place or trail that is quiet, where you can be exposed to nature.

- Take the opportunity to breathe deeply and walk upright.

- Use the time to pray and meditate. This is an ideal time to talk to the Creator.

- Try to appreciate nature during your walk.

- Drink plenty of water after each walk.

- Apart from your daily walk, consider taking the stairs instead of the elevator. Do not get upset if you cannot park close to the grocery store. Walking a little distance can only help. Use every opportunity to be active.

S—SELF-CONTROL

"Do you not know that your body is a temple of the Holy Spirit, who is in you, whom you have received from God? You are not your own; you were bought at a price. Therefore honor God with your body." I Co 6: 19, 20

Self-control is vitally important. Self-control can apply to many areas of your life including time, ingestion of toxic substances (e.g. tobacco, alcohol), speech, and appetite. With obesity, the biggest hurdle may be appetite, but with others it may be with our tongue. If you lack self-control with regard to appetite, it can lead to the following troublesome set of circumstances: you start to overeat, usually the wrong kinds of foods → your quality of sleep deteriorates due to obstructive sleep apnea and heartburn → you become chronically tired with concentration and memory problems → it becomes difficult to exercise since you are always exhausted → you gain more weight due to the lack of exercise and become grouchy, depressed and want to eat even more. Your self-esteem starts to suffer. Everything spirals downward. Unfortunately, this is a common scenario. If you need help with self-control, I recommend the following:

- Recognize that your body is not your own but God's. Realize that when God's spirit fully dwells in the temple (which is your body, mind, and brain) it is very difficult to remain overweight, stressed, or to be spiritual dysfunctional.

- Be aware that if *self* is not in control, something else is. Identify what **is** controlling you.

- Do not hesitate to ask God for help.

- Eat nutritious foods. These foods can be restorative and delicious. With a little effort and planning, you can find foods that are healthy, support weight loss and are tasty. By following all of God's health laws, the brain and mind are able to function well. Often, simply following God's natural health laws, the problem of self-control can be taken care of automatically.

- Obtaining self-control may take time and effort, but God can help to lessen your struggle.

- Giving up should never be an option! If you make a mistake, start over and keep trying.

T—TIME

"There is a time for everything and a season for every activity under heaven."
Ecclesiastes 3:1

Time is one of the greatest gifts we have. Time can be very profitable and beneficial if used wisely. When it comes to restoration, time is important. When you commit to fitness and take all of the appropriate steps toward reaching that goal, at that moment the battle is more than halfway won. Getting on the right path is more important than reaching ones destination because given time you will succeed by the grace of God.

God's timetable is different than ours. He may choose to take longer than you would prefer, or He may take care of your problem much sooner than you could have ever imagined. Either way, God is the master coordinator and knows what He is doing. Although God's timing is different than yours, His timetable is undeniably better. Healing takes only as long as it takes for **God's** agenda to be completed. All you need to do is exercise patience and trust. With respect to time, I recommend the following:

- Make the proper lifestyle changes now. Do not procrastinate as it will only become harder to change with the passage of time.

- Be patient, always.

- It is more important to commit to change than to focus on the time it takes to reach your goal. You *will* get there!

- Focus on the present when it comes to the necessary health changes you need to make. But also envision your eventual future state of wellness.

O—OBEDIENCE

"As obedient children, do not conform to the evil desires you had when you lived in ignorance." 1Peter 1:14

Obedience is crucial when it comes to restoration. Unfortunately, disease does not discriminate between willful disobedience and one that stems from ignorance. The end result of disobedience to natural health laws is the same. Because illness is a personal matter, it is imperative that each individual take responsibility for learning everything necessary regarding their health. Disobedience may prevent total wellness from occurring.

The first place to start is with obedience to God's laws, spiritual, physical and mental. God's all inclusive laws are designed to provide optimal health in all areas of your life. Adam and Eve were given instructions on the type of foods to eat that would allow proper functioning not only of their body but also of their mind. This would allow them to effectively commune with their Creator, the most important aspect of wellness.

As with disobedience pertaining to other rules, there are consequences, sometimes severe ones, when it comes to health. The consequences may be immediate or they may be delayed, and insidious in their onset. It is never too late to start obeying God's laws. It is also important to realize that:

- Obedience is a safeguard against self-destruction and harm.

- Health laws come in one package that must be kept in their entirety.

- Obedience involves trust and confidence that the health laws given are beneficial. Natural laws are restorative. However, never confuse nature with the God of nature. Only God is infallible and omnipotent.

- Obedience to proper health laws is voluntary but only temporarily so. You can choose to obey now or be forced to obey later.

- Obedience to health laws is synonymous with health promotion, health maintenance and disease prevention. None of these are passive acts. Effort is required.

- Obedience to health laws may be viewed as an investment for future wellness.

- By full obedience to God's law, you can go from being morbidly obese to reaching your ideal body weight, naturally.

R—REST

"There remains, then, a Sabbath-rest for the people of God"
Hebrews 4:9

Rest in all forms is important. Without adequate rest, full restoration is impossible. When resting or relaxing, one can recuperate physically, mentally, and spiritually. There are in fact several types of rests:

1. Sleep. Sleep is very important because it allows reparation of your body from the wear and tear encountered throughout the day. During deep sleep, important hormones are released such as growth hormones and leptins which are important in metabolism and weight management. The brain, which never shuts off, is at least able to rest during deep sleep since blood flow to the brain and its metabolism slows down considerably. With proper sleep, one is subsequently invigorated and mentally refreshed. Sleep deprivation can cause or exacerbate a variety of problems including mood and stress which can complicate the battle against weight loss. With regard to sleep, I recommend:

   a. Get at least eight hours of sleep daily. The exact amount will vary between individuals.

b.   Go to bed at least a couple hours before midnight. *An hour of sleep before midnight is worth several hours of sleep after midnight.*

c.   Avoid going to bed on a full stomach, in a noisy environment, or after consuming caffeinated products. All of these can interfere with the quality of sleep.

d.   Invest in a comfortable mattress.

e.   It is easier to get a good night sleep after a busy and physically active day than one during which you were idle.

f.   If you have difficulties falling asleep, contact your physician. Instead of settling for a sleeping pill, try to find out the underlying cause of your sleep disturbance.

2.   Relaxation. Proper relaxation can be a powerful agent to combat stress. Stress is a common etiologic problem in obese individuals and should always be addressed. The mind cannot remain in overdrive constantly. Without adequate relaxation, chronic stress, mood dysfunction and anxiety symptoms may develop, not to mention cognitive difficulties. Somatic symptoms can also become evident if you consider that stress produces various chemicals that affect the organs of the body (brain, gut, lungs, heart and other muscles). When it comes to weight loss, stress must go!

3.   Sabbath rest. Just as we require daily rest, the Bible teaches the necessity of having a weekly rest called the Sabbath. This is a type of rest that provides spiritual renewal, and to which a blessing is attached (read Exodus 20: 8-11).

A—ACCOUNTABILITY

"Nothing in all creation is hidden from God's sight. Everything is uncovered and laid bare before the eyes of Him to whom we must give account."
Hebrews 4: 13

When it comes to obesity, you must first understand your condition. Genes play a role in obesity, but so do environmental factors that you *can* control. Do not hesitate to take responsibility for your actions when you are at fault. Poor diet, a stressful lifestyle, lack of exercise, chronic anger and other negative emotions can all be the culprits. Acknowledging your shortcomings is the first step toward restoration. Only after the root of your problem has been identified can the appropriate steps be taken to prevent or correct the problem.

You do not need to be a medical doctor to understand the basics of health and illness. The fact that obesity can lead to many problems is common knowledge. You should empower yourself by learning about everything that pertains to your health and safety. It is in fact a solemn responsibility to understand the steps necessary to ensure your fitness. I recommend the following:

- Identify the cause of your obesity.

- Look closely at the following factors:

  - Your diet (quality, quantity and timing).

  - Your stressors.

  - Your relationships with other people.

    - This includes family members, relatives and friends.

    - Your enemies.

  - Your spiritual life.

    - Are you humble and forgiving?

    - Do you trust in God?

    - Is there is a sense of purpose in your life?

  - Your self-image/self-worth/self-esteem.

  - Your level of activity.

    - Are you sedentary?

- Decide to take action *today*.

  - Seek appropriate help.

  - Address any lifestyle and nutrition issues that may be present.

Never procrastinate when it comes to your health!

T—TRUST IN GOD

"Trust in the Lord with all your heart and lean not on your own understanding; in all your ways acknowledge Him, and He will make your paths straight."
Proverbs 3: 5, 6

Trusting in God is the pivotal point of the RESTORATION model. There are several reasons why it is important to trust in God:

- He created man, and knows the source and solution for all our infirmities.

- God is omnipotent (all powerful). He can recreate, remodel, repair, and remove our illnesses. He can speed up your metabolism, even if your genes dictate otherwise. You must do your part though and follow His health instructions.

- God has *your* best interests in mind, all the time. He is the only one that truly understands what your best interests are.

- By placing your complete trust in God's ability to help you, you manifest faith, which is imperative when it comes to healing.

- You must have faith since "without faith, it is impossible to please God" Hebrews 11:6

  - The components of faith are:

    - **F—FEAR** the Lord, shun evil and live uprightly.

    - **A**—Do not be afraid to **ASK**. Be bold in your requests.

    - **I**—Be **INSISTENT**.

    - **T**—Have unwavering **TRUST** in God, and respect his **TIMETABLE.**

    - **H**—Only then can you expect **HEALING** and total RESTORATION

Trusting in God has an element of surrendering your will to God. That process is healthy and can provide peace. When healing occurs, it is important to give praise to God and to be thankful. If you really have faith, you can start the praise and thanksgiving *before* the healing is manifested.

I—INSIGHT

"For I know my transgressions, and my sin is always before me."
Psalm 51:3

Insight, hindsight and foresight should all go together. It is your responsibility to consider possible mistakes you have made in the past, assess the present, and take informed steps to ensure future wellness. Be your own medical detective. It is a fact that most obese individuals have problems that are related to lifestyle and nutrition. Many of these conditions are entirely preventable, and can be managed naturally. Understanding the source of your problem thoroughly and taking steps to correct it is **vital**. It is important to *want* to lose weight and to be prepared to take the appropriate steps required. If you lack insight, you can always ask God and He will be only too happy to give it to you.

O—OPTIMISM

"So do not throw away your confidence; it will be richly rewarded."
Hebrews 10:35, 36

Optimism is always important. With optimism comes positive anticipation and hope. According to the RESTORATION model, you can be optimistic because the ultimate source of healing is God. He is certainly not lacking in healing power, wisdom, mercy, or understanding. Armed with this belief, you can step forward and engage in the activities that are necessary for your weight loss to occur. If you are not optimistic, you will not put forth the effort necessary to get off to a good start towards weight loss. If you are not optimistic and you should happen to fail the first or second time, you will easily give up. If you are not optimistic, every obstacle, real or imagined will appear colossal. Each accomplishment will seem insignificant. By being optimistic, it allows you to set a goal. Optimism is the path that can lead you to success.

N—NUTRITION

"Then God said, 'I give you every seed-bearing plant on the face of the whole earth and every tree that has fruit with seed in it. They will be yours for food.'"
Genesis 1:29

Eating nutritiously is perhaps the natural law that is most often broken by individuals with an obesity problem. As far as weight management, few foods are neutral. There are foods that can promote weight gain, while others foods have the opposite effect. Beverages are the same. Some beverages, like water, can quench your thirst, cleanse and detoxify your body, and not add one calorie to your weight. Others, such as caffeinated sodas, can cause you to store unneeded calories, weaken your immune system, cause headaches, and still not properly quench your thirst. The goal of nutrition should not only be to satisfy hunger, but also to meet the daily requirements of the body. When this is done, there should be no unhealthy cravings, weight gain, water retention, or other types of disturbances commonly encountered in obese/malnourished individuals. We should eat to live healthy and productive lives instead of living to eat and then be at risk for death-producing illnesses.

I recommend the following:

- Drink approximately 8 glasses of water daily. More specifically, the amount of ounces equivalent to half of your body's weight in pounds.

- Eat plenty of raw fruits and vegetables daily. Among other things, they contain enzymes, fiber, antioxidants, minerals, vitamins, water and perhaps thousands of phytochemicals that are as yet unnamed.

- Avoid dairy products. Substitute it with soy/rice based products.

- Avoid caffeinated beverages and foods (chocolate) and red drinks.

- Eat low glycemic foods.

- Avoid food additives like MSG, nitrates, and Aspartame/NutraSweet.

- Avoid sweets. They are your number one enemy, even above fat.

- Consider taking nutritional supplements such as antioxidants, essential fatty acids, glyconutrients, minerals, phytochemicals, and vitamins. Natural supplements are a better and safer way to support weight loss, compared to weight loss drugs that have the potential to cause severe adverse effects.

If you are confused and overwhelmed about which foods are best to eat and which ones may be contributing to your weight problem, just consider the following:

- You can never go wrong with foods that are fresh and raw. The best examples are fruits and vegetables that contain enzymes to help you digest what you eat and other essential nutrients such as vitamins, minerals, antioxidants, phytochemicals, phytosterols as well as fiber and water. All these substances help support weight loss while promoting health.

- You should be cautious of foods that are *decorated and treated* with unsafe chemicals and dyes but devoid of useful nutrients.

    - There is a difference between:

        - Fresh potatoes versus potato chips

        - Apples versus apple pie

        - Carrots versus carrot cake

If you eat foods that are overly processed, this means that you are malnourished. You may be obese and still malnourished, if you are eating the wrong types of food. Being malnourished can intensify or directly cause a variety of physical and mental health problems. It is impossible to lose weight effectively without addressing nutritional factors thoroughly.

13

Conclusion

If you are obese and are not enjoying optimal health, there is hope. God is the ultimate healer, and He can help you. He has provided simple health laws and natural *tools* that are in nature to assist you. These health *tools* are abundant, readily available, inexpensive, safe, effective and restorative (i.e. vitamins, minerals, phytochemicals, etc.). Using God's health laws, which include proper nutrition, hydration, temperance, stress-free living, and spiritual renewal, you can experience total wellness.

While finding the right exercise program, buying the right healthy foods, and taking the right dietary supplements are all important for ultimate success to be reached, a total spiritual renewal is necessary first. You need to acquire strength and will power. You need to be optimistic. In my case, as a health conscious physician, I knew just what I had to do and was constantly plagued by the saying *"physician heal thyself"*. There was a gap between my knowledge and the actual application of that knowledge. It was not until I placed matters in God's hands using the principles of the RESTORATION model that I was able to get on the path toward success that resulted in my losing 100 lbs after years of struggling. More important than the weight I lost, was the realization that I was entirely transformed, mentally and spiritually. I was totally restored! This can also be your experience, by the grace of God.

"Praise the Lord, O my soul and forget not all his benefits. Who forgives all your sins and heals all your diseases, which redeems your life from the pit and crowns you with love and compassion, which satisfies your

desires with good things so that your youth is renewed like the eagles." Psalms 103: 2-5.

GLOSSARY

Abortifacient—causes an abortion.

Adipocytes—fat cells.

Arachidonic acid—an amino acid that enhances inflammation in our bodies. It is found in meat, meat products and eggs.

Aromatherapy—the inhalation of volatile oils in the treatment of a health condition.

Ayurveda—a 5000 year old system of mind-body medicine. It originated in India. It uses herbs, nutrition, meditation, yoga and massage. Some cases of metal poisoning have been reported from contaminated ayurvedic medications with arsenic, lead, and mercury.

Binge eating—a condition where a person eats a large amount of food in a short period of time.

BMI—body mass index. The BMI is determined by dividing an individual's mass in kilograms by their height in meters squared.

Capsaicin—comes from chili and red peppers. It may cause mild weight loss.

Carminative—a substance that assists with the removal gas from the intestinal tract.

Carotenoids—are present in dark-green leafy vegetables and orange and yellow fruits and vegetables. Good sources of carotenoids are carrots, sweet potatoes, and peaches. Carotenoids are precursors of vitamin A.

Chromium—an essential trace nutrient found in meats, fish, whole grains, cheese and vegetables.

Citrus aurantium—bitter orange, which contains small amounts of alkaloids. It is believed that citrus aurantium acts similarly to the ephedra alkaloids.

Emmenagogue—assists with menses.

Garcinia cambogia—contains hydroxycitric acid (HCA). HCA has been shown to decrease food intake, body weight gain and body lipid content. These studies have not been reproduced in human subjects.

Ginkgo biloba—is an antioxidant. It enhances neurotransmission.

Glucomannan—is another water-soluble fiber that leads to weight loss without being part of a prescribed diet.

Guar gum—a water-soluble fiber that reduces hunger and weight more effectively than water-insoluble bran fiber.

Homeopathy—uses dilute preparations of natural substances to cure illness. The belief of Homeopaths is that "like cures like".

Inositol—a substance found in vegetables and liver.

Iron—a mineral found in dried fruit, leafy greens, strawberries, nuts, fish, and poultry.

Leptin—A hormone secreted by adipocytes involved in weight control.

Magnesium—a mineral present in dark green vegetables, legumes, nuts, seafood, and whole grain cereals and breads.

Naturopathy—emphasizes prevention of illness. There are 3 accredited schools in the US.

Reike—a Japanese form of healing where energy flows from the healer to the patient/recipient.

Rubefacient—a substance that causes the skin surface to become red once it is applied. It works by causing vasodilatation of the superficial blood vessels.

Selenium—a mineral that supports the antioxidants. Dietary sources of selenium are yeast, nuts, fish, and sunflower seeds.

Zinc—a mineral found in lean red meats, peas, beans, and whole grains.

BIBLIOGRAPHY

Alternative medicine and the perimenopause an evidence-based review. M. Taylor. Obstetrics and Gynecology Clinics of North America. Volume 29(3), 555-73, September 1, 2002.

Behavior Modification in the Treatment of Obesity. M. Hyder, BA, K. O'Byrne, BA, W. Poston, MPH, PhD, J. Foreyt, PhD. Clinics in Family Practice. Volume 4, Number 2, June 2002.

BrainRecovery.com Powerful Therapy for Challenging Brain Disorder. David Perlmutter, MD. The Perlmutter Health Center. Naples, Florida, 2000.

Childhood obesity. Child and Adolescent Psychiatric Clinics of North America. C.M. Morgan, M. Tanofsky-Kraff, D.E. Wilfley, JA Yanovski. Volume 11(2): 257-78. April 1, 2002.

Child to adult socioeconomic conditions and obesity in a national cohort. Internal Journal of Obesity Related Metabolic Disorders. C. Power, O. Manor, S. Matthews. Volume 27(9): 1081-6. September 1, 2003.

Commonly used herbal medicines in the United States: a review. S. Bent, MD and R. Ko, PharmD, PhD. American Journal of Medicine. Volume 116, Number 7, April 1, 2004.

Contribution of pathogens in human obesity. N.V. Dhurandhar. Drug News & Perspectives. Volume 17(5), 307-13, June 1, 2004.

Decreased energy levels can cause and sustain obesity. D. Wlodek & M. Gonzales. Journal of Theoretical Biology. Volume 225 (1), 33-44, November 7, 2003.

Earlier onset of puberty in girls: relationship to increased body mass index and race. P. Kaplowitz, E. Slara, R. Wasserman, S. Pedlow, M. Herman-Giddens. Pediatrics 2001. Volume 108: 347-53.

Editor's Overview of the Conference on Preventing Childhood Obesity. S. Lederman, PhD, S. Akabas, PhD, B. Moore, PhD. Pediatrics. Volume 114, Number 4, October 2004.

Emphasize Fitness Over Weight Loss, Expert Says. K. Johnson. Internal Medicine News. October 2004.

Etiology and Natural History of Obesity. G. Bray, MD. Clinics in Family Practice. Volume 4, Number 2, June 2002.

Fat poisons livers of the obese. United Press International. June 15, 2004.

Herbal Cures for Common Ailments. Jim O'Brien. Globe Digests. 1997.

Herbal preparations for obesity: are they useful? D. Heber, MD, PhD. Primary Care; Clinics in Office Practice. Volume 30, Number 2, June 2003.

Herbal Remedies and Children: Do They Work? Are They Harmful? Alan D. Woolf, MD, MPH. Pediatrics. Volume 112, Number 1. July 2003, pp.240-246.

Glyconutritionals: Consolidated Review of Potential Benefits. Glycoscience & Nutrition. July 6, 2001.

Liposuction doesn't change metabolic problems. Anthony J. Brown, MD. Reuters Health. June 16, 2004.

Medical Complications of Obesity. J. Whitman, MD. Clinics in Family Practice. Volume 4, Number 2, June 2002.

Obesity Gene Therapy Target Found. United Press International. June 17, 2004.

Obesity in Children and Adolescents. W. Brown, MD, FAAP, K. Sibille, MA, LMHC, L. Phelps MD, K. McFarlane, MD. Clinics in Family Practice. Volume 4, Number 3, September 2002.

Obesity may soon be leading cause of preventable death in US. Canadian Medical Association Journal. Volume 166, Number 5, March 5, 2002.

Obesity risk doubled for kids of obese moms. Merritt McKinney. Reuters Health Information. July 7, 2004.

Obesity: Special Features. G. Bray. Journal of Clinical Endocrinology and Metabolism. Volume 89, Number 6, June 2004.

Obesity, Weight Gain, and the Risk of Kidney Stones. Eric N. Taylor, MD, Meir J. Stampfer, MD & DrPH, and Gary C. Curhan, MD, ScD. JAMA, January 26, 2005. Volume 293, Number 4.

One signal makes stem cells into fat cells. United Press International. June 22, 2004.

Overeating tied to drug use withdrawal. United Press International. July 9, 2004.

Paediatric Neurology. Edward M. Brett, MD, DM, FRCP. Churchill Livingstone. 3rd Edition, 1997.

Pediatric Neurology: Principles and Practice. Kenneth F. Swaiman, MD. Mosby. Second Edition, 1994.

Pharmacotherapy for the obese patient. R. Carek MD, MS & L. Dickerson, PharmD, BCPS. Clinics in Family Practice. Volume4, Number 2, June 2002.

Prevalence of Overweight and Obesity among Adults with Diagnosed Diabetes-United States, 1988-1994 and 199-2002. MS Eberhardt, PhD et al. MMWR 2004; 53: 1066-1068.

Surgery may benefit severely obese teens. Will Boggs, MD. Reuters Health. July 6, 2004.

The Antioxidant Miracle. Lester Packer, PhD & Carol Colman. 1999.

The genetics of obesity. C. Damcott. PhD, P. Sack, MD, A. Shuldiner, MD. Endocrinology and Metabolism Clinics. Volume 32, Number 4, December 2003.

The Psychologic Correlates of Obesity. M. McGuire, PhD, R. Jeffrey, PhD, S. French, PhD. Clinics in Family Practice. Volume 4, June 2002.

The Role of Physical Activity in Obesity Management. S. Paluska, MD. Clinics in Family Practice. Volume4, Number 2, June 2002.

<u>Treating and Preventing Obesity through Diet</u>. Practical Approaches for Family Physicians. G. Gans PhD, MPH, LDN, J. Wyli-Rosett, EdD, RD, C. Eaton, MD. Clinics in Family Practice. Volume 4, Number 2, June 2002.

<u>Treatment choice is ultimately the patient's</u>. M. Fleming, MD. American Medical News. Page 19, October 4, 2004.

About the authors

Drs. Jean-Ronel Corbier and Michelle Corbier are Christian physicians who are interested in wellness using an integrative approach. They are board certified in neurology with an emphasis on child neurology and pediatrics respectively. They felt the need to broaden their perspective regarding health and disease. Dr. Jean-Ronel Corbier's desire to be broad-minded medically started at Michigan State University where he decided to enroll concurrently in medical school and a graduate program in health and humanities. The latter program gave him the opportunity to work with health practitioners who use a more holistic approach in treating patients. Dr. Jean-Ronel Corbier completed his neurological training at the University of Cincinnati and Children's Hospital of Cincinnati, with additional neurological rotations at Johns Hopkins and the Mayo clinic. In particular, their Christian faith and strong spiritual background have enabled them to incorporate biblical principles in the treatment of patients using a model they developed called the RESTORATION model. This model is dynamic, natural, comprehensive, etiologic-based and curative. Dr. Jean-Ronel Corbier has a medical practice in Montgomery, Alabama. Dr. Michelle Corbier also completed medical school at Michigan State University. She left private practice to help her husband manage his office and to home school their son, Jean-Michel.

0-595-34708-8